White Oak Dental PLLC
2600 North M-52
Stockbridge, MI 49285
517-851-8902

TOOTH TRUTH

A Patient's Guide to Metal-Free Dentistry

© 1995, 2000 by Frank Jerome, D.D.S.

Published by:
New Century Press
1055 Bay Boulevard, Suite C
Chula Vista, CA 91911
(800) 519-2465
(619) 476-7400
www.newcenturypress.com

Library of Congress Card Number: 00-103323
ISBN 1-890035-13-0

D1060054

This book is dedicated to:
My wife Linda, for years of help,
Dr. Hulda Clark for her never-ending
search for the truth;
Dr. Hal Huggins, who sounded the trumpet to
begin
the battle to end mercury fillings; and
All the patients who have suffered from
dentistry's toxic materials and treatments.

DISCLAIMER

Unless presented otherwise the opinions and conclusions expressed in this book are mine and mine alone. They are based upon observations that I have made while practicing my profession. Please understand that I cannot be responsible for any adverse effects believed due to the use of information in this book. You should be guided by your own dentist or physician, whom you may wish to educate by providing a copy of this book.

FOREWORD

The severe toxicity of mercury has been known for centuries. The dental profession still continues to promote mercury silver fillings and the use of other toxic therapies.

The human body's natural ability to heal itself and the immune system has been under attack by not only environmental pollution, but also by procedural pollution from dental and medical professions with the use of toxic drugs, chemicals, root-canal therapy, radiation and excessive surgeries. Rather than take leadership in protecting people from poisons, they actively support and condone the addition of chemicals, such as fluorides in the environment.

Recent research has shown that in Idiopathic (no apparent cause) Cardiomyopathy (disease of heart muscle), mercury is 22,000 times higher than normal. Despite this shocking discovery, standard cardiology does not seem interested.

To avert this double whammy from the dental and medical professions, a paradigm shift must be made to procedures which protect the body's natural ability to heal and which naturally enhance the immune system.

Perhaps in this litigious and economically pressurized world it is impossible for the average professional to admit, "If I am not part of the solution to disease, I may be part of the problem." Patients must demand better treatment. If the patient's mouths are "toxic dumps," physicians cannot aid the patient in fighting degenerative diseases. Dr. Frank J. Jerome's book, Tooth Truth, is a must read for patients and professionals.

I certainly hope that this book will help raise awareness to the dangers of "modern" dentistry. As we enter the 21st century, it would be a good time to leave toxic dentistry behind.

James P. Frackelton, M.D.
Past-President, American College
for
Advancement in Medicine
24700 Center Ridge Road
Cleveland, OH 44145

INTRODUCTION TO UPDATE

I wish I could tell you things have gotten better since I first wrote this book, but the opposite is true. The economics is still driving the system, not health; this is to be expected, as economics drives everything. If the economics were based on biocompatibility first, there might be a chance for improvement. If people better understood what really is happening to them rather than blindly trusting their dentist, excuse me, their dental care provider, they would have a chance to protect themselves.

With the state of dental materials being in a state of flux, it is difficult to make hard and fast recommendations. A few rules still apply: The more difficult the procedure the more likely there will be a bad result; natural tissues are better than manmade materials; biocompatibility should be a top consideration, and no tooth is worth damaging your immune system. If you use these four rules, you can save yourself much grief.

To help people keep up with the changes requires applying the principles in this book with what is available at your dentists' office. A new material may come along that satisfies all four principles the day after the book goes to print (highly unlikely). The answer to keep you current is the Internet. As a service to people who are seeking the most current information please check out our website at **www.dentistry-toothtruth.com**. If you are not on the Internet yet, it is available free at most libraries. Do not be afraid of it, as it is easy to learn, and you do not need to know about computers to use it. Please do not let any fear of technology stop you.

Hundreds of people have asked us to refer them to a dentist near them who does the same thing we do. For years we tried using various lists of dentist who are mercury-free and have taken the same seminars we have. Later the people who went elsewhere called back with one complaint or another. It became clear that since we do not know specifically what any other dentist might do, we cannot give any referrals. Perhaps in the future we will have the ability to refer people to dentists with similar practice philosophies and skills. Instead of referring, we encourage people to learn how to know what is happening when they go to any other dentist.

We are all a bit lazy and want to trust our care providers to know things so we will not have to think for ourselves; that is not in our best interest. So, as painful as it is, you must know what is going on. This book is a shield of information to prepare you to understand what a professional might advise you to do. If their opinion is different than ours, you need to tools to help judge what you hear. Do not be afraid to ask questions on anything you do not understand. It is your body and your money, so you have every right to choose what is in your best interest and no one else's.

INTRODUCTION

We seek the truth, and will endure the consequences.
Charles Seymour
Statement made while president
of Yale University [1937-1950].

This book will discuss disturbing information. Most people have accepted whatever treatment their dentist has recommended without question. No one wants to learn that what dentists have had implanted in their bodies is the source of growing levels of toxic substances that can wreck their immune system and destroy their most precious gift, good health.

Most of us expect good health, even while doing almost everything we can to undermine it. We eat too much and rest too little. We actively seek vices that can slowly or quickly destroy us. We take unnecessary risks, as if we earn points for foolhardy behavior. The last thing any of us wants to know is that there is another major source of ill health that is to some degree affecting all of us right this minute and will probably worsen every day. It is easy to turn a deaf ear to this information, but ignorance does not make it safe.

Many people fondly remember when we could smoke and drink without worrying because we were not fully aware of the devastation these habits cause. Somehow it seems that these habits only became dangerous once we knew they are dangerous. Maybe it is the recklessness of youth that blinds us to the consequences of our acts. Maturity carries a price, and that price is taking responsibility for our own health.

We can no longer hide behind the assurances of those people who say they will save us from our follies. It does us little good to wait until we are a few months from death to get our habits of decades corrected. If we are to give ourselves the gift of a life of good health, we must find out the hidden daggers stuck in our backs by our health professionals. We all know of stories of misdiagnosis, the inaccurate prescription, or the wrong leg being amputated. While we wish to trust our fate to others, we really know it is our own responsibility to take care of ourselves and our families.

Dentistry is not exempt from doing more harm than good. The history of the use of toxic mercury is just the tip of the iceberg when it comes to the ills dentists have caused their patients. The list of other toxic materials is long, but it does not stop there. The actual procedures dentists use carry high risks of damage not only to the teeth that they are trying to help, but to the health of the whole body.

While we may not want to know what these problems are, we must learn because there is no one else to do it for us. This book is a warning to every person that there is much danger every time they enter a dental office. If you do not learn how to stop this damage, the road back to good health may not be possible. Once you understand the risk you will be better able to protect yourself. So reluctant or not, read and learn.

CONTENTS

1

WHAT'S THE PROBLEM?

Metal-Free Dentistry

"The Future of Dentistry is Metal-Free."
Murray Vimy, D.D.S.
Past president and co-founder of The International Academy of
Oral Medicine and Toxicology (IAOMT)

There is an ongoing battle among dentists about the risks of using mercury in fillings but this book greatly widens the debate by challenging the use of all metals used in dentistry. It is important that you understand the differences between mercury-using dentistry, mercury-free dentistry, and metal-free dentistry.

Dentists who use mercury generally do the procedures they were taught in dental school and follow the company line as espoused by the American Dental Association. In contrast, mercury-free dentists have come to question the validity of some of what they were taught in dental school and question the validity and honesty of the ADA. But the dentists who practice metal-free dentistry must question everything, including the validity of every material, procedure and concept.

Metal-free dentists must rethink the purpose, the technique, and the outcome of every dental procedure and the dental materials used: Learn to find and treat causes, not just symptoms; look for side effects from what has been done in the past; and determine what can be done to correct these side effects without causing more problems. This is a very difficult task because they must not only do non-damaging treatments but try to overcome previous damage caused by toxic dental materials and harsh techniques. Because they know the damage that can occur, they believe prevention of the original problem is the safest course and that if anything must be done, it has to save as much of the original tissues as humanly possible.

Seeing Problems

Many mercury-using dentists claim that if there were problems they would have seen them in their patients. But to see something you must look. For example, if someone told you your backyard was full of animals, you might run to the window and look out. Not seeing any lions or tigers or bears, you might turn to the person and tell them they are crazy. But if you took a shovel, a screen sieve and a magnifying glass and began to look under the surface, you would find huge numbers of animal species living very active lives. The problems caused by mercury and other metals are also hidden. You must look a bit deeper, but when you do, there is a lot of activity going on.

Another reason dentists do not see a major reaction when they place a mercury filling in a patient is that the patient usually has many fillings already present. If a patient has ten mercury fillings, will placing an eleventh filling cause immediate changes? Probably not, but if they had no mercury fillings and a dentist placed eleven all at once, changes would be much more apparent.

It is rare that so many fillings would be placed in unfilled teeth, but it is not rare for mercury-free dentists to remove eleven fillings

4

over a short period of time; when they do, the patients routinely tell of improvements in their health and their feeling of well-being.

That is why mercury-free dentists see what mercury-using dentists do not. If mercury-using dentists would follow the same procedures, they would see the same results. Unfortunately, very few mercury-using dentists ever get the chance to remove mercury in such a manner that would get a positive response from a patient. With the current political atmosphere in dentistry, the mercury-using dentists will continue to look out the window and not see nothing.

The Attitudes Of Dentists

Dentists are mostly honest and dedicated people. It is quite possible that they are familiar with every problem discussed in this book but their first inclination may be to ignore or dismiss what is said. They may also see many ideas they had themselves, for example, questions about materials and procedures they may have raised as students but that were ignored or put off by instructors. It is possible they may see many things with which they agree. It will be the first time they have seen so many aspects of the practice of dentistry challenged.

The dental profession, through its leadership, has generally ignored or denied the truth. Therefore, this book has been written directly to the consumers, their patients. It is hoped that consumers will decide with their dollars what type of materials and procedures they really want once they are better informed. It is time to re-examine what dentists do and for better choices to be made.

Coming Changes

Readers should be aware that the forces against mercury are growing throughout the world. The tidal wave of change coming from outside the dental profession will force it to change. Dentists still have a chance to direct the wave of change but not to stop it. But time is limited. Unless there is a radical change in dentists' attitudes, the change will be thrust upon them by governments, lawyers, and consumers. Regardless of dentists' personal feelings, they cannot ignore these forces that are, at this moment, forging the future of dentistry. The problems with mercury fillings are only the tip of the iceberg of the problems surrounding dental materials and procedures.

You might ask, "If my dentist has heard about all of these problems and in his opinion they do not need to be considered, then why should I worry about them?" Well, first, you need to consider that your dentist may be wrong. If so, what is the impact on your life and the lives of your family? Secondly, their motivation is colored by the economics of the profession. While most professionals believe themselves to be above basing their decisions on money, the reality is their decisions are all economically based.

The next question is, "Does money unduly influence their treatment decisions?" Hopefully, the answer is, "No, not usually, but there are exceptions." Dentists are in the business of delivering dental services. The more services they can provide and the more profit in those procedures, the better off the dentist will be financially.

The dentist will try to show you that the benefits of a proposed treatment outweigh the costs. However, the chances are that the benefits of almost all dental procedures do not come close to being of value to the patient. The standard for everything that is sold is "let the buyer beware"; it is sound advice in the dental office, too.

Learning Your Options

Critics of this book will say that a dentist who suggests that patients should get the metals out of their mouths is just using it as a marketing ploy. While it is true that anything can be manipulated for the wrong reason, the information in this book will help you tell when you are being manipulated. Patients must also beware of dentists who say they are getting your mercury fillings out, but who may be putting something worse in their place.

Use the information in this book to protect yourself from ALL dentists. The book's purpose is to increase your ability to detect the truth from the nonsense. Getting rid of metals, infected teeth and all the other results of misdirected dental treatments is really "anti-dental work." The true value of dentistry is to prevent problems, not repair them after they occur.

Dentists who do not place mercury fillings believe that prevention is the best treatment. They do not believe that simply putting fluoride in our water will solve the decay problem. While they do not want to do any unnecessary treatments for you, they have to do something to help you get rid of damaging dental work already present and its influences on your health. They are trapped into making the best of a bad situation knowing that any treatment is less than perfect. They try to correct patients' problems with the least amount of treatment possible.

The economics of a dental treatment is best shown by the example of how a crown or cap is sold to a patient. Every practice management course stresses the need to do more crowns because they are the most financially beneficial procedure that is done in the average dental office, generating the most money per hour. A reasonably skilled dentist can generate $300 per hour and up doing crowns compared to $150 per hour doing cleanings or fillings. Doubling your income is a strong motivator!

Optional Treatments

It is common knowledge among dentists that over 95 percent of all dental treatments are optional. If 95 percent of any business is optional, don't you think there has to be a lot of selling going on? It is economically very important for the dentist to motivate patients to undergo these optional treatments, but for whose benefit and at what price? You must be informed as to the realities of these optional treatments, so you can make informed decisions as to what you want done and how it will affect the rest of your body. The purpose of this book is to show dental treatments for what they are, "the good, the bad and the ugly." The dental treatments your dentist may recommend may not be what you need to maintain or regain your body's health. You must be able to tell the difference.

Defending Yourself

The current major controversy in dentistry is over the use of mercury in dental fillings. Unfortunately, there are many other types of damaging dental materials and procedures. It is time for a complete review of the entire profession of dentistry. It is time for everything to be re-evaluated, with only the best materials and the least damaging procedures being kept. It will be a traumatic time for dentists, but it is the patients who must be thought of first. This book is the patient's "self-defense" manual.

It is hoped that this information will result in a consumer re-evaluation of current dental practices supplying the information needed to ask the hard questions and demand specific answers. In turn, this attitude will force dentists to be more aware of the effects their treatments have on their patients. It is also hoped that individuals who have "dentist-caused problems" will be able to find their cause and have it corrected, so they may begin to heal.

As a patient, you have been "trained" to do as you are told. This blind belief in the altruistic (selfless) behavior of dentists, as well as other professionals, has left people vulnerable to manipulation and abuse. It is time to think for yourself. You must re-educate yourself to be able to separate the truth from the half-truth and lie.

This book is to show you the many ways to look at your dental health and to caution you that the dentist's way may not be the best way for you. No professional likes to have his patients or clients challenge what he says and dentists are no exception. But it is your health at stake, and you need to be prepared to challenge any treatment that may be against your best interests. The attitude patients must learn is that you are responsible for your own health. Being informed is your best defense.

I Don't Want To Be A Dentist!

People, who after years of health lessons in school, countless magazine articles, TV ads and visits to dentists, seem to know very little about their mouth. They know what a tongue is, but go blank when it comes to taste buds. They know the white things are teeth and that some of them are called molars or back teeth and some are front teeth. They probably have heard of eye-teeth (canine or cuspid), but not everyone knows which ones they are. It is not really that complicated and if you are to get the most out of this book, it is worth a bit of trouble to educate yourself. If you go to a dentist and do not have any knowledge of the basics, you are at his mercy and must accept what he says. Deferring to a dentist is what got people in the condition they are in now.

If the dentist neither understands your concerns nor what needs to be corrected because he is blinded by his training, you must understand. You must have an idea of what materials and treatments you have had placed in your mouth so you can understand what it will take to replace them. If you do not participate in planning your treatment, you can easily be worse off when the dentist is done. Ignore this information at your peril.

Basics

You are born with the potential for two sets of teeth; twenty baby teeth (which will not be discussed) and thirty-two adult teeth. The adult teeth are divided into two arches with sixteen teeth in the upper arch and sixteen teeth in the lower arch. Easy so far?

There are eight teeth on each side of each arch which makes four sets of eight teeth or quadrants; upper right, upper left, lower right, and lower left. Each side of the arch is the mirror image of the other side. You can more easily understand by looking at the illustration (Fig. 1.1).

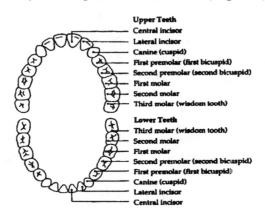

Upper Teeth
Central incisor
Lateral incisor
Canine (cuspid)
First premolar (first bicuspid)
Second premolar (second bicuspid)
First molar
Second molar
Third molar (wisdom tooth)

Lower Teeth
Third molar (wisdom tooth)
Second molar
First molar
Second premolar (second bicuspid)
First premolar (first bicuspid)
Canine (cuspid)
Lateral incisor
Central incisor

Tooth Names

Figure 1.1

Each tooth of the eight matches the corresponding tooth in each of the other arches. In other words each quadrant of eight has a front tooth; therefore you have four front teeth, two up and two down. The last tooth in each arch is a wisdom tooth; therefore you have four wisdom teeth and so on. Each of the eight has a name. The first one is Fred, then Ethel, Lucy, Rickie—just kidding. The real names are central incisor, lateral (side) incisor, canine, cuspid or eye-tooth, first bicuspid, second bicuspid, first molar, second molar, and third molar or wisdom tooth.

The common way for people to look at teeth is front teeth and back teeth. The first two of each eight are front, the two

11

incisors, central and lateral; they are called incisors because they incise or cut. Since each quadrant has two front teeth, you end up with eight front teeth, four up and four down. These teeth are positioned flat to the front so they are considered to run side to side. The next tooth, the cuspid, stands by itself at the corner of the mouth. The arch turns at the cuspid from being side to side in the front to being lined up front to back along the side. Think of the cuspid as a corner post. It is a very strong tooth and corresponds to the mighty fangs in the animal kingdom. It has only one point or cusp, which is where it gets its name cuspid.

The remaining teeth are back teeth. The first two are bicuspids because they have two cusps. The last three are molars, which have about four cusps and are called molars because they mill or grind food.

Are you bored yet? Maybe just a little. Stick with it just a bit longer. The first teeth that come in around age six are the central incisors followed by the lateral incisor and the first molar, which is also called the six-year molar. Nothing much happens until age eleven when the second molar, which is also called the twelve-year molar, comes in. In most Americans the wisdom teeth lack necessary room and are extracted around age 18. This leaves us with 28 teeth, which would be very adequate if they could all stay that way. Unfortunately for us and fortunately for dentists we insist on damaging our teeth.

Each tooth is made of three distinct parts. The enamel, the dentin, which makes up the majority of the tooth, and the pulp chamber and root-canals, which are the source of nutrients and waste disposal. You really knew that, didn't you?

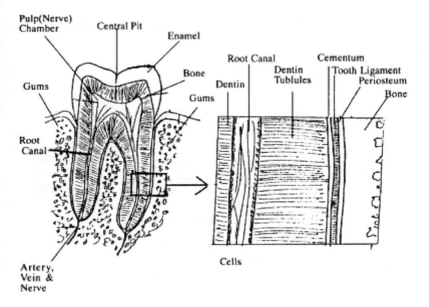

Anatomy Of A Tooth

Figure 1.2

There are two layers which are small and technical. The first is the cementum, which covers the outside of the root just as the enamel covers the top or crown of the tooth. The cementum is very thin and not visible without a microscope but does play some important roles. (See Figure 1.2.)

The final layer is the ligament which holds the tooth to the bone. Teeth are not connected directly to the bone but are held by the ligaments which connect the cementum to the covering of the bone (periostem). The presence of the ligament is what allows orthodontist to straighten teeth and lets us sense the hardness of the foods we are chewing.

13

Dentists look at teeth as five-sided boxes with a root on the sixth side. They size fillings by the number of sides or surfaces that are involved; one surface, two surfaces, etc. (See Fig. 1.3). When too much of the tooth is involved or if there are three or more surfaces involved in a filling, dentists are taught to think of putting

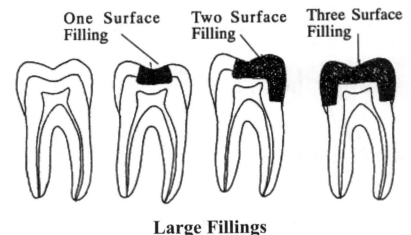

Large Fillings

Figure 1.3

on a total cover for the tooth called a crown. It is not uncommon for some dentists to recommend crowns on teeth with one or two surface fillings. Such dentists are dangerous to your health.

If the decay gets too large or deep, the pulp chamber becomes infected. The body protects itself by forming a sac at the end of the root as shown in Figure 1.4. This is when dentists do root-canal therapy. Another example is shown in Figure 1.5 where a tooth with a three-surface filling has been treated with root-canal therapy. The inside of the tooth has been cleaned, shaped and then filled. This example shows a post which can be added for strength.

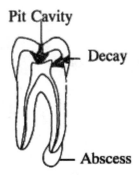

Figure 1.4

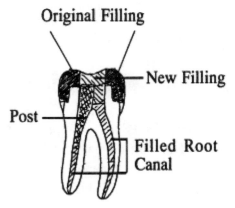

Figure 1.5

Figure 1.6 shows a cross-section of a badly broken down, root-canal-treated tooth which has been rebuilt using a post and core buildup and a crown. These procedures are done to give strength to the weak remaining root. Figure 1.7 is the same tooth as Figure 1.6 with all the dentist-added materials removed. When viewed in the mouth, the tooth in Figure 6 would look like a nice solid tooth but in reality only a small portion of the original tooth is left and it is very weak and brittle.

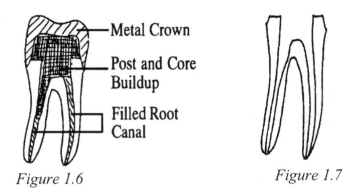

Figure 1.6   *Figure 1.7*

This description gives you a quick lesson in how you got where you are today. The rest of the book will try to tell you why certain work was done and your alternatives.

Avoiding Bias

In his Indianapolis Star newspaper column, John Shaughnessy wrote of his use of the "Kid Principle of Fairness and Logic." He said, "When doubt or controversy arises in a situation, people choose a lot of different ways to determine what's fair and logical.... Stated simply, the principle holds that if a situation doesn't seem fair or make sense to a child, there's most likely something unfair or illogical about it.... But, generally, if children think through a situation, they'll reach a conclusion that's simple and eloquent in both its fairness and its logic."

There are other ways to say this: What would an "honest man" say about the situation? The legal profession uses the "reasonable man rule." Our grandparents would use the term "common sense," which is usually quite uncommon. All of these are ways of reasoning to come to a conclusion based on the facts presented, and not anything else. Those "elses" include biases due

16

to friendship, family, money, and power; lying ("false witnessing"); cheating; Biblical "coveting;" "saving face;" and "covering your rear end with paper," to name a few. You can find examples of any and all of these warped methods of reasoning every day in the newspapers.

It is often said there are three sides to every controversy: your side, my side, and the truth. It is not possible to write without some bias sneaking in. But it is the intent of this author to try to tell the unvarnished truth and let the "chips fall where they may." By applying the "Kid Principle of Fairness and Logic," along with the "honest man," the "reasonable man," and "common sense" concepts, this book tries to tell the truth.

In the recent movie, "A Few Good Men," during a courtroom scene between Tom Cruise, the lawyer, and Jack Nicholson, the tough Marine colonel, the lawyer shouts, "I want the truth!" The Marine colonel snarls back, "You can't handle the truth!" Can YOU handle the truth?

It seems that very few of us want to know the "unvarnished" truth, at least, not on a regular basis. We usually settle for our illusions and hope for the best. Even after we hear any truth, we tend to return to our illusions. But we do owe it to ourselves to at least see the truth every now and then. Maybe over the years we will move our illusions closer and closer to that truth.

The Progression Of Dental Treatment

The progression of dental treatment refers to the increasing amounts of treatment done to patients as the natural oral tissues break down and are replaced with dental materials. We are all familiar with this phenomenon.

People start out with a full set of teeth and by the time they die, most have lost many teeth with the rest of their teeth full of dentists' handiwork. Twenty-five percent of Americans are without any natural teeth when they die!

It is actually said that Americans have the best dental care in the world. The question that comes to mind is, " Why do we need so much dental work?" We should have the best, but need the least. The lack of healthy teeth is a symptom of many dietary problems we cause ourselves. Many poor countries are full of people with beautiful healthy teeth, the likes of which American dentists have never seen.

To give you a better idea of the possible steps in this progression, here is a typical story of a person's dental experience. It begins with a child getting his first permanent teeth. By age eight he has 24 teeth, half baby teeth and half permanent teeth. The most common decay begins forming on the first molar (also called the six-year molar because it comes in at age six). The cavity (dental caries) is in the most common location, the pits and grooves on the top of the tooth. The cavity is found at age ten and a small mercury filling is placed.

During the teenage years a lot of soda drinking and other nutritional shortcomings, combined with a lack of thorough daily cleaning, results in decay on the side of the tooth. Another, larger mercury filling is done. At age 18, the four wisdom teeth (or third molars) are removed by an oral surgeon.

Eight years later at age 26, an area of decay undermines a coner of the tooth and a cusp breaks off. Now there are three sides of the tooth damaged by decay. A dentist tells the patient that the tooth is weak and covers it with a gold crown. Two years later the tooth abscesses, meaning it dies and becomes gangrenous. The tooth is "saved" with a root-canal. The patient is now in his late twenties.

After another ten years the gums and bone around the tooth weaken due to damage from the original abscess, which never fully healed. The tooth has to be extracted. The patient is now 39. The dentist suggests that after healing, a bridge be placed to fill the space and prevent the other teeth from moving.

Since the price of gold has gone up, the dentist recommends a porcelain-covered, nickel bridge. This three-tooth bridge has a crown on the second molar (the 12-year molar) and one on the second bicuspid (the smaller tooth in front of the missing tooth). The pontic fills the place of the missing first molar. The bridge is then cemented into place.

Twelve years go by and there is a further weakening of the bony support of the 12-year molar, the crowned back tooth (one of the bridge abutments). It becomes loose and has to be extracted. Only the front crown (the other bridge abutment) is left. Now no molars are left. The dentist suggests a chromium and cobalt partial. The dentist says, "This will help maintain your ability to chew." The patient says, "Go ahead. I have insurance!" The patient is now 54.

Later, the patient finds out he has high blood pressure and begins to take medicine to lower it. His physician also tells him to quit his 36-year smoking habit. The medicine makes his mouth dry, but the physician does not worry about its effects on the mouth, because after all, the medicine may be preventing a heart attack. The mouth thus becomes more acidic because of a lack of saliva to dilute the acids.

The patient does not like having a dry mouth since he has to speak to the public in his job. The acids make his mouth taste metallic. So the patient begins to chew gum, but the sugarless types stick to his partial. He finds a gum that does not stick to his dental work, but it is not sugar-free. His mouth may feel better while it becomes even more acidic. An occasional bag of lemon drops seems to stimulate more saliva. These sugar sources create more acids, which attack the teeth under the partial.

Meanwhile, the patient continues smoking because his efforts to quit have been too stressful. The attacks of the acids combined with the effects of smoking on the gums and bone badly damage the other teeth. The dentist refers the patient to a periodontist (gum doctor) for surgery.

After the patient's gums are in better shape the original dentist repairs or crowns other teeth. The patient is now 62. He has finally quit smoking but is still under stress as his job has been eliminated, forcing him to take early retirement. Since he does not draw enough money from his pension, he must take another job.

The combination of all these stresses causes the patient to begin to grind his teeth in his sleep. The pressure this grinding puts on the remaining teeth is too much in their weakened condition and further bone loss occurs. It becomes difficult to chew because the teeth are tender. Certain foods, the more nutritious ones, are eaten less frequently. The patient does not want to take extra vitamins and minerals because, as many often say, "I don't like to take any pills!" The bone loss rapidly accelerates. Several more teeth are past saving and more are weakening.

Eventually, the patient becomes tired of all the pain and hassle his teeth are causing him. He tells the dentist that he wants the rest of his teeth removed and "plates" (a complete set of dentures, commonly called false teeth) made. The dentist makes the dentures, removes the remaining teeth, and puts in the dentures. In the next 6 to 12 months, after healing is completed, a reline (reprocessing technique) is done to make the dentures fit better. The patient is now 71.

Sixty-five years after the first permanent teeth came in, the patient has no natural teeth left. The various dentists and the patient have worked closely together as the patient's mouth was slowly destroyed by both poor health habits and too much dental treatment.

Many readers will recognize their parents in this example. Many may even recognize themselves. While this dental deterioration is "normal" in Americans, it is not natural for a human to end up toothless or with a mouth full of metal. As you go through this book, you will see where other choices could have been made by both the patient and the dentist.

This book is to help you know the options so you can stop this downward progression. More importantly, it will show how various dental treatments and materials may actually be the cause of the decline of your general health.

Dentists may complain that this example is not that of an "average" patient. They may say that it may have been true before twenty years ago, but their patients' dental health is better now. While there has been a trend for more people to keep more teeth longer, it is far from the level it should be. There are still many people whose teeth have become so damaged that they have lost them all before they are 25. There is much room for improvement. The trend is moving away from prevention and toward more elaborate dental work; for example, a hot new dental area is implants.

Unfortunately, this movement away from prevention is causing the majority of the work done by dentists to involve the repair of previous work done by dentists. It is not that the original work was not done well, although that is very common. Dental work wears out, gets used up, breaks down or new problems arise next to it. These problems are considered the "natural" progression of the breakdown of the teeth and their supporting structures through use and misuse; this is partly due to the improper ways people take care of their teeth through their daily care and nutrition.

Dentists pay little attention to prevention. They promote fluoridation and feel they have done their duty. They tell you to brush and floss or they have someone else tell you, such as a dental hygienist or a TV commercial. They may suggest you quit smoking or eat less sugar.

Twenty-five years ago some dentists made an effort to move into nutritional counseling and improving their patients' total eating pattern. They met with resistance because this effort made dentists consider areas outside the mouth. It was also difficult for them to get paid for what patients perceived as only talk, not action. Patients expect to pay dentists only when they do something to a tooth. Patients also did not want to change current habits for long-term gain. Delayed gratification is not common in America, and the movement lost momentum in the 1980's. But many dentists involved in the prevention movement continue to work toward better total health for their patients. As leaders in the mercury-free dentistry movement, they are questioning many of the traditional dental materials and procedures.

Dental Practice Limits

Dentists are careful not to exceed the areas of practices covered by their license, avoiding any treatments that might be considered medical practice. This mindset severely limits the thinking of the profession and separates dentists and physicians more than they are in most other countries. Instead of thinking of themselves as physicians who specialize in the oral cavity, dentistry concentrates on mechanical repairs. Dentists are so preoccupied with the repair of teeth, in fact, that they cannot see the damage these procedures do to other areas of the body. The unspoken agreement with physicians is that dentists will not look outside the oral cavity and physicians will leave all mechanical treatment in the oral cavity to dentists.

Many problems that seem to defy routine medical treatment may be due to effects of dental materials. For example, it matters little what a physician does to treat depression if it is caused by mercury from the patient's fillings.

We are all aware that depression is a major problem in America. It seems as if half the population is on Prozac. Yet most people are unaware that depression is a common side effect of mercury exposure. Since the vast majority of Americans have or had mercury fillings, could there be a connection? Would a large number of people stop being depressed if their mercury fillings were "properly" removed? Dentists who remove mercury fillings routinely see patients become less and less depressed. However, it is considered unethical for a dentist to suggest that a patient have his mercury filling replaced for any reason except poor condition of the fillings. To do otherwise--treat depression by removing mercury fillings--would be considered by other dentists to be practicing medicine.

It is not just the patients who lack the necessary information; the majority of dentists have little or no knowledge of the toxic effects of their dental materials. As students, they endured the courses on dental materials and as practicing dentists, rarely if ever go back and read the current research. They rely on others, particularly the biased American Dental Association (ADA), to tell them what they can use. Those that speak out against mercury and other toxic materials are denied access to the major dental media and assemblies. No debate is going on within the ADA between the pro-mercury and anti-mercury groups because the pro-mercury group tends to "stonewall" the issue, only responding when they have no other choice. When the issue is presented, the pro-mercury group presents both sides, purporting to be unbiased but are careful to avoid a direct challenge. Therefore, patients cannot rely on most dentists to give them the information they need to make choices that can affect their health for the rest of their lives.

A good example of how the ADA stifles debate on this issue occurred a few years ago. After "60 Minutes" aired a segment on the toxic effects of mercury fillings on patients in December, 1991, the ADA and the pro-mercury dentists fought with every lie and half truth they could find to continue their use of mercury fillings. They issued pro-mercury position papers to every dentist in the ADA to pass out to their patients. Even when Dr. Gordon Christiansen, a popular researcher, stated that mercury is the most toxic filling material, they paid no attention.

The fight for more biocompatible materials started 15 years ago and since then, has gained enough grass-roots strength to reach national attention. The battles are being joined on every front: research, legal, federal government, media and public opinion. But most important will be how the patients themselves feel about what is being done to them without their knowledge. When all the truth is out, people are going to be very angry about the decades of mistreatment. But anger will not bring back lost health.

The Future Of Dental Education

The ADA News reported on February 6, 1995 on the conclusions of a two-year National Academy of Sciences Institute of Medicine on dental education. This report is very important because most dentists closely follow their training throughout their entire career, which the committee recognized. The ADA News said, "The report issues 22 challenges for change for education and profession alike, presenting the status quo as a path to stagnation and decline." If only new dentists follow these new recommendations, it will take over 30 years before change is fully realized; that means dentists already in practice must also accept new ideas and learn to challenge the status quo.

The report urged a closer integration of dentistry with medicine because there needs to be "more medical management of oral health problems." The report argued "One problem with oral health services (indeed, health services generally) is limited evidence about the effectiveness of many preventive, diagnostic, and therapeutic interventions." That statement can be interpreted to say that dentists are doing wrong things for the wrong reasons and even the things that they say are preventative may not really work.

The report also stated that "just as the effectiveness of a dental treatment cannot be assumed, neither can the effectiveness of practice guidelines." So these researchers believe that not only are some dental procedures lacking in effectiveness but so are the guidelines which are imposed on dentists. That is a pretty heavy statement and it is not being leveled by maverick dentists but by a blue ribbon panel of dental educators. This report must make you wonder if any of those ineffective procedures have been done on you.

Symptoms

"You can never treat enough symptoms to correct the cause."
Dr. Ted Morter, Jr. D.C. Author and Past-
President of Logan College of Chiropractic

Our society is symptom-oriented. We believe the symptoms are the problem, not the solution. To understand how symptom-oriented we as a culture are, write down every TV commercial you see in a two-hour period. You will see commercials for gas, stomach pain, allergies, gum disease, bad breath, hemorrhoids, yeast infection, incontinence, athlete's foot, body odor, and sweating, to name a few of the common ones.

Almost every commercial about health problems is concerned only with the symptoms the product can relieve, ignoring the underlying cause of any of these problems. Have a fever, take an aspirin. Have heartburn, take an antacid. The trouble with this emphasis on symptoms is that we forget what they really mean. We believe that the symptoms are the disease, which leads us to many false assumptions about how to take care of ourselves. Symptoms can tell us two things: first, they can act as a warning system, such as when we feel pain and secondly, they are the outward effects of the immune system as it fights any invading foreign material, be it germs or pollen. We should use these symptoms to monitor our health to see if our defense systems are working, not to tell us what drugs to take to suppress them.

If you sprain your ankle, the first thing you want to do is "reduce the swelling." But swelling is your body's defense to protect the ankle; it forms a natural splint. The pain is also a symptom we want to eliminate, but it also has a purpose in keeping us from using the damaged ankle. When we block the pain receptors of the brain with drugs and take something to "make the swelling go down," we are defeating our body's defenses. We tend to use the damaged ankle too soon, so it does not fully heal. The ankle may then become permanently weak and more vulnerable to respraining.

As you can see, altering or masking symptoms for convenience may carry a high price. Consider the treatment for a common cold. By treating cold symptoms, we allow the invading germs to greatly increase their numbers and turn a three-day cold into a lingering illness. Any bacteria, viruses or yeast that invade our bodies and are not destroyed may become so strong and well-hidden that they can never be completely destroyed. From then on our immune system has to work constantly just to hold these invaders in check.

The Common Cold

If our body is attacked by a cold virus, we get a runny nose. The purpose of our body secreting excess mucous (the runny nose) is to create more of a barrier to attacking germs and to flush them out of our body and gives us needed time to develop antibodies specific to the invading germs. Because we view the runny nose as the germs winning over the body rather than the body fighting the germs, we want to eliminate the symptom, the runny nose. So we take an anti-histamine, which dries up the runny nose. We think we have "shown those germs a thing or two," but what we really did was remove our first line of defense. Now the germs can easily penetrate our body in large numbers that overwhelm our immune system, which has not had time to prepare the antibodies. The cold gets a big head start and, therefore, it takes us much longer to recover.

Do you know people who complain how long their recent cold lasted? Have you heard people say how a cold settled in their chest and they could not shake it? You probably hear these complaints all the time, and may have said them yourself.

Other Examples

Another classic example is our treatment of fever. We believe that fever is caused by germs and should therefore be reduced. People think reducing the fever will make them get better. We may have gotten the idea from those old movies in which the country doctor sat up all night with the sick child. Just at the right moment "the fever broke" and we knew the child would survive. With drugs we can "break" the fever any time we wish and save sitting up all night. It seems the thing to do because we are warned about not letting the fever get too high. If it keeps going up to 106 degrees, we could suffer "brain damage." And who wants to have brain damage?

So what is the truth? Fever is a symptom that the immune system is working. The invading germs do not cause the fever; the body creates the fever to fight the invaders. The body is in charge, not the germs. The temperature goes up to 102 degrees when the invader is a bacteria and 104 degrees when it is a virus. The higher body temperature increases the body's defenses as it weakens the invader. The body knows what it is doing; the fever does not exceed our involuntary control. In a very few instances, such as meningitis, an infection around the brain, the body fights so desperately to kill the invader germs that the temperature reaches 106 degrees. This rise is indeed serious and is why the temperature needs to be taken. When the temperature climbs to 105 or above, the person needs to be in a hospital to protect him from heat stroke and dehydration, but not to lower the temperature the body has chosen to protect itself. The "fever breaks" when the body has overcome the infection. The body will reduce its own temperature when the need has passed and does not need outside help.

What happens if you take something to reduce a fever? The truth is that you are helping the invading germs, be they bacteria or viruses. When the body's temperature is artificially lowered with drugs, the body cannot fight back enough to destroy them. The invaders are able to penetrate deeper into the tissues and may become a chronic infection. In America we have many people suffering from such chronic infections, ones that never leave.

Many children, for example, were damaged by being given aspirin to reduce their fevers and developing Reye's syndrome. It took a long time to figure out the cause. Very few people use aspirin to reduce fever now. Unfortunately, they still take other drugs. They learned the wrong lesson!

Another example is the high incidence of death by pneumonia. The cause of this fatal infection is hidden in our bodies for years, waiting for our immune system to be preoccupied with another emergency so it can multiply. Before our immune system can respond, our body may be overwhelmed. "The operation was a success, but the patient died."

We are reluctant to let nature take its course. We are too busy. We have to get to work and do not want to be inconvenienced by being hot and sweaty. So we take a pill to reduce the fever and push on. Eventually, we may pay a high price in ill health for being so hard on ourselves.

Symptom Misuse In Dentistry

How does this treatment of symptoms rather than underlying causes apply to dentistry? Many patients will have a symptom of a problem that they are unable to ignore even after using different types of pills. Some leftover antibiotics (if antibiotics are taken correctly, there will never be any pills left over!) will hold down an infection for a while, but it usually returns much worse. Pain killers available over-the-counter will control a lot of pain. Taken long enough, these pills may give the body enough time to cause the pain to leave because the infection begins to drain. The infection will not ever go away completely, but many people are satisfied if they have avoided a trip to the dentist's office.

In TV commercials, people are encouraged to buy a topical anesthetic to ease denture pain from ill-fitting dentures. However, the pain is a symptom, a warning of a problem. The gum-numbing topical anesthetic only helps for a short time. The answer lies in getting the denture adjusted so it fits. If the irritation is allowed to continue, deep cuts can result, cuts that may in time become painless because the brain has become insensitive to the warning signals. This chronic irritation may cause thickening of the gum tissue and even cancer.

In another example many patients will see a black area develop on a tooth. They know that it is decay but think they will wait for a more immediate symptom, like pain, before seeing a dentist. They think it is not much of a problem because it does not

30

hurt. Unfortunately, by the time it does hurt, there is usually infection involved and an abscess is forming. The bacteria are usually invading the body via the blood. What had been a small problem has become a major one. Tooth loss or worse will follow.

Treating Symptoms

Are dentists better at seeing the cause of problems rather than the symptoms? Not really. Tooth decay is a symptom that dentists treat as a disease. They think the cure is a filling. Does filling the cavity change any of the causes that allowed it to form? No. If none of the causes are corrected, would you expect more cavities to follow? Yes, and they do. The use of mercury is one way that dentists actually cause more harm by treating the symptom rather than the underlying problem, because mercury itself is a cause of illness. If a dentist treats your symptom, the cavity, with a material, mercury, that causes disease, are you really any better off? We need to stop the decay that causes cavities by stopping the cause of decay, poor diets. We must also rid ourselves of mercury and other toxic dental materials to prevent further damage to our bodies. Why repair a tooth with a material that can damage the kidneys and brain?

We must learn to look for the causes of problems and stop treating only the symptoms. Treating symptoms never solves anything; it usually makes matters worse. Any short-term gain in comfort will be paid for in long-term problems and a lowering of the immune system functions. We must learn that healing is a return to health, not a pill that will control 12 symptoms. In fact, most symptom control lets us abuse ourselves more than we could without it. The symptom control stresses our natural healing ability, sometimes so much that it cannot recover. The answer is to stop abusing our bodies and let them have enough time to heal. It may seem to be the harder way to go, but in the long run, we will be much healthier.

Oral health is not a mouth full of gold crowns, not teeth refilled with the best composite fillings ever done. Oral health is enjoying life with a full set of whole, healthy teeth in healthy bone that is covered with healthy gums. When we make that the goal of dentistry, we will be addressing the causes, not the symptoms.

"Cookbook" Dentistry

A dental educator once taught that there are only two basic concepts to remember to be a successful dentist: "The front teeth have to look good and the back teeth have to be pain-free." (Anonymous) He said if these two rules are followed, the patients will be happy and the dentist will make a good living.

Dentists like to have an obvious answer for every problem they face. When they look at an X-ray and see a cavity, they know if they follow standard procedures, they can repair the damage, collect a fee, and everyone will be happy. Dentists want the standards of care to be fixed so every dentist will provide about the same services.

Dentists like to know what comes next. If a tooth needs a large filling, dentists know that they should do a crown. If the tooth dies, dentists know that they can do a root-canal. If the tooth is visible, dentists know that they can cover the crown with white porcelain. These criteria are straightforward "cookbook" dentistry. No thinking is required, just follow the recipe.

If a dentist starts saying that any of those standard services are wrong, the rest of the dentists get angry. They do not like dentists who "make waves" because it rocks their boat, and boat rockers are not appreciated anywhere. The rule is, "You have to go along, to get along." Thus, any dentist who challenges the standards of care is ignored. If such a dentist is too outspoken, he is attacked. If possible, his license to practice dentistry is threatened or revoked. The average dentist feels much more threatened by an outspoken dentist, who raises questions about what is sound dental practice, than by a dentist who does poor dental work but keeps his mouth shut.

Comrades, Not Competence

Once there was an old-time dentist still practicing in the 1970's who treated patients without taking X-rays. He did not use any numbing, either. He would drill a little and put in a filling. Patients loved him because he was considered painless and they did not get "shots." As you can imagine, a lot of decay was left under fillings. Without X-rays, he never saw decay between teeth. The other dentists said nothing about his treatments, even though they knew that they were far below the "standard of care." When finally asked, these dentists said he was not "too bad," plus he was "such a nice guy." Unfortunately for this dentist, he died soon after. Hopefully, all his patients were then better served by other dentists.

This dentist was not a threat to his fellow-dentists because he did not challenge their work and likewise, they did not challenge his. A dentist who challenges the majority is considered a danger. A dentist who tells the public the things that are told in this book may be considered a traitor to the profession even if every word were true. No group likes to have their dirty laundry aired in public! Unfortunately, no change will happen without the public demanding better treatment. Countless attempts have been made to correct these matters from within the profession, but nothing has changed in 20 years, except for the worse.

Dr. Hal Huggins

One noteworthy example of a dentist who challenged standard procedures is Dr. Hal Huggins, who was in the forefront of the current anti-mercury movement, giving lectures at dental meetings across the country during the 1970's. Most of the dentists who lead the anti-mercury groups now were started in this new direction by Dr. Huggins.

Then suddenly, he was no longer at any meetings. It seemed that he was "making too many waves." According to reliable accounts, someone told meeting organizers that if Dr. Huggins was on the program, the ADA would withhold official recognition. Dentists would get no continuing education credits for attending any of the lectures at the meeting. That was enough to end Dr. Huggins lecturing at any ADA-approved meetings, effectively keeping the anti-mercury message away from the majority of dentists.

Dr. Hulda R. Clark

Dr. Hulda Clark has sparked a growing debate on the way diseases are treated. Her one-woman crusade to help people escape the archaic methods of many medical practices has taken root. She now has an ever-growing group of supporters all over the world. Her claim that the body is self-healing, once we can clean up the body of toxins, bacterial invasions, poor nutrition and parasites, is echoed throughout the literature. She has joined earlier voices against the toxic effects of dental materials. The debate on dental materials has begun. The manufacturers will listen to the demand to make dental materials biocompatible, as more patients demand such materials from their dentists. The problem is that there are sick people needing help today.

Dr. Clark advises that cancer patients need to have their filled teeth removed, most difficult in America where there is no consensus that this is a valid treatment. In the not too distant past physicians advised Americans to have their teeth out to stop arthritis. Teeth are not the cause of arthritis, although some of the dental materials could have been involved. Still, untold numbers of Americans lost their teeth.

Some dentists believe that once a tooth has suffered years of large fillings and is contaminated with bacteria and metal oxides, it should be extracted. Most patients resist having such teeth removed and other dentists are quick to attack a dentist who even takes out abscessed teeth. This attack makes it politically dangerous for dentists who are trying to help those people who follow Dr. Clark's recommendation.

It is difficult to develop a consensus and it may take a generation or even two. There should be options for patients who are willing to follow Dr. Clark's advice but today there are not.

As her research develops, other options will hopefully emerge. Since there have been many developments since the first *Tooth Truth* was published, it is best to check her website for additional information. Our website **(dentistry-tooth truth.com)** will also try to post any new information concerning Dr. Clark's research.

It is also important to note that Dr. Clark has strong views on the use of commercial toothpastes. While toothpastes are not covered in this book, people need to be aware that there are many alternatives. A good case can be made for using baking soda, although Dr. Clark has more recommendations you may wish to consider. It has long been known that if a patient properly brushes, they will do a better job with just water than with commercial products. The foaming action of toothpastes limits most brushing to just seconds. We will try to offer some options on our website.

Inflexibility

If you show this book to a dentist who "knows" what the normal treatment should be, he may be very angry. He may tell you that this is all lies, that you should not believe such "junk." He may feel threatened because if he accepted the ideas in this book, he would not know what to do. All the nice "cookbook dentistry" he has been following throughout his professional life is shown to be wrong; that would be a hard idea for any professional to accept. Dentists will resist this information even when it is obvious to everyone else.

Unfortunately, most dentists will try to convince you to doubt what is written here. They tend to resist new methods because change is always threatening. If information about such methods comes from patients, they will resist even more. Stand your ground. Do not get any treatment done if you cannot get it done right. If you are confused, wait. Do not be bullied into a treatment that you feel may not be safe. The only way dentists will stop using mercury fillings is if every patient says, "No!" It is better to wait than to undergo some treatment that may harm you or that might have to be redone.

Just remember, as a patient, you do not have to allow a dentist to treat you. If all patients refuse to allow toxic treatments, or treatments of symptoms rather than underlying causes, dentists will have to change or find another line of work. As a patient, you have the power to stop toxic treatments. It is time for the dentists to get a new cookbook!

Death Through Dentistry

"In their addiction to the slogan 'save the tooth,'
dentists increasingly lost the patient."

> Martin H. Fischer, M.D., Professor of Physiology at the University of Cincinnati, Author of Death & Dentistry (1940)

It is a common belief among dentists that they do not do anything that kills patients. Many chose dentistry over medicine because they do not want to deal in life-and-death situations. But the truth is that dentists do contribute to the early death of patients and may lead to their deaths directly.

One of a dentist's biggest fears is having a patient die in the chair. Such a death is infrequent, but dentists are careful to avoid taking risks. For example, patients with serious health problems are referred to specialists for procedures that carry risks, such as extractions. Even oral surgeons will hospitalize some patients so that they will be able to pass on their care to a physician if the patient suffers any health crisis. All these precautions are prudent.

If a patient has a life-threatening crisis in a dentist's office, the dentist will call for assistance. If the patient actually dies, he is given CPR until the paramedics come; that way he will be considered alive when he leaves the office. If he is DOA at the hospital or dies later, it is better than a headline saying, "Patient Dies in Dr. Blank's Office." Just the thought of this happening gives dentists the chills. Even though immediate deaths from dental treatment are rare, the damage done by toxic dental materials and procedures to the immune system is severe and can further weaken organs and organ systems.

Trouble After Treatment

If an older patient has dental work done, feels poorly for several days after, then dies of a heart attack, will the dentist be called? Or will the dentist read about this patient in the obits and think, "Mr. Smith died, and we had just finished all his work. That's too bad. I wonder how it happened?" The dentist will not consider that any of his treatments may have triggered the crisis that led to the patient's death. The family may know about the dental work, but likewise never think that there is a connection. They would find other reasons that explain the death: He was old; he had a weak heart; he had been getting worse for years.

Other Considerations

Dr. Michael Ziff states in his book *The Missing Link?* that dental work can trigger a heart attack by stressing a damaged heart through anxiety alone, but it can also do so through materials. For instance, mercury can cause "blood vessel constriction and subsequent hypertension within minutes after exposure."

In other, even more subtle, ways dental treatment can contribute to an early death. For example, an infection from an extraction or a root-canal could challenge the immune system so that a person could go into a health decline that ends in death even years later. What if the immune system is so challenged by a dental treatment that a mild case of the flu turns into pneumonia? What if treatment for a gum infection, such as the new techniques in which antibiotic cords are placed under the gums for long periods, causes a drug allergy to develop? Or what about a group of highly drug-resistant bacteria that may develop due to mercury fillings that could tip the balance from recovery to death? Other effects, such as cavitations (remnants of infections from previous tooth extractions) can cause serious damage in areas of the body remote from the mouth.

The extent of damage done by dentists is just beginning to be acknowledged in the current American dental literature. Medical studies and foreign dental literature, on the other hand, have been describing these problems for over sixty years. As research goes on, it will become increasingly apparent that dentistry carries much higher risks than you have been led to believe.

Informed Consent

Informed Consent is a legal concept meaning you should be informed of the risks, as well as the benefits, of a procedure before it is done. Physicians have used it for years, mostly to ward off legal problems. Once a patient is told of possible negative outcomes and agrees anyway, they have no reason to complain if the results are less than hoped for.

There has been a movement to have dentists use Informed Consent forms, so that patients will know the effects of the materials used. Part of the rationale behind this movement is to try to stop the use of mercury. It is reasoned that if a patient was told that toxic mercury was going to be used, they would say no.

It is true that many people will reject mercury fillings once they know what they are made of and what can happen as a result of such fillings That is one reason dentists do not call them mercury fillings. To avoid using the word "mercury," dentists call them silver fillings or amalgams.

It is also true that most people will use whatever the dentist suggests without thinking. Even patients who have had their mercury fillings removed by one dentist may have other mercury fillings replaced by another. They report that the dentist said it was the only material they could use, or they said that mercury fillings were better or cheaper. Such reports show that the major influence is not facts but the power of the dentist's recommendation.

Reclaim Your Rights

It is time for patients to reclaim their rights. The right to choose is always the patient's. It has been easier for people to let the "professional" choose for them than to become informed. You should never give up your rights, even in times of crisis, especially in times of crisis. The tendency is always for the person who is making the decisions for a patient, to choose what is in their best interest, not the patient's best interest.

Informed Consent at least puts the facts down on paper so they are before the patient and shows that there are serious problems with most dental materials. The negative effects of dental materials have been kept from the public to avoid rejection of the treatments recommended by dentists. Many negative effects are just accepted by the dentists as normal risks, just as smokers accept shortness of breath. This book brings all the risks into the open so both the patient and the dentist can see how what is placed in the mouth can affect the whole body.

California, which usually leads the nation in new ideas, has begun requiring Informed Consent forms for dental materials. California has 20 percent of the U.S. population, therefore 20 percent of the dental patients are covered by this ruling. Hopefully, other states will follow.

Appendix I is an Informed Consent form you may copy for personal use. This form will allow you to be told of possible side effects that are now being denied and may be used for any procedure or material. In dentistry, because so many of the treatments are toxic, it is wise to have an Informed Consent form filled out for each treatment. Dentists will not happily fill this out, but it is in your best interest to know what can happen. It is in the dentist's best interest to be accurate when the form is filled out. Omission of potential side effects would leave the dentist legally exposed.

Remember, this form may save your life. Do not ignore its ability to protect you from harm. The form will warn a dentist that he must be concerned about the possible effects of his treatments on your overall health.

2

HOW TO FIND THE TRUTH

A truth is a new sense, for with it comes the ability to see things we could not see before—and things that cannot be seen by those who do have that new truth.

> Dr. Weston Price famed author and former chief researcher for the ADA

There are many stories of corruption and concealment in our newspapers. You read the stories, but how are you to know who is telling the truth? Individuals lie, cheat, and steal for many reasons. Organized groups do it for power and money. If you want to know where the truth is, follow the money because whoever gets the money is lying.

"Whistleblowers," at least those who tell the truth, generally have more to lose than anyone else. Yet they take this risk because their sense of what is right has been violated. Most people tolerate a minor corruption of values, but when it becomes so great that it affects everything a person does, that person must "speak out or get out!" Attacks on whistleblowers are so common that the federal government has laws to protect individuals who come forward to expose corruption. These laws are helpful, but they cannot fully protect the truth-tellers who will always pay a price. For many the price is death. We are all familiar with stories of "stool pigeons," who sometimes wind up "missing" or dead. Many people consider such people as "tattletales," a name for kids who tell adults about other kids who are breaking the rules.

That while tattletales are regarded badly does not mean they were not telling the truth. In fact, it is because they tell the truth that they are such a threat. If they were lying, tattletales could be confronted with the truth and be dismissed. But if what they say is the truth, the people in power do not want it exposed.

The nice thing about telling the truth is that you do not have to remember what you said. Liars always have to remember what they said so they do not trap themselves in a lie. We have many expressions to describe this, such as Sir Walter Scott's, "Oh, what a tangled web we weave, when first we practice to deceive!" and "the truth will (come) out." Knowing this is the nature of truth (and lying) helps the police get suspects to confess their crimes. Unfortunately, if the policing organization itself (in this case, the ADA) is telling the lie, this makes it much harder to untangle the truth from the lies.

The Long View

Historically, the truth comes out, but it can take fifty years or more. If you are the one hurt by the lies, fifty years may be too long to wait. If mercury and other dental materials and procedures are hurting millions of people, fifty more years means unnecessary misery and harm on a huge scale. And worse, more people are added every day. The cost in damaged and ruined lives is beyond calculation or understanding. Shame to all those who dare perpetuate these lies for their own profit, either out of ignorance or to hide their guilt.

This book touches on hidden truths in many areas other than dentistry; each deserves attention to expose the reality behind the image. We believe too easily the lies of those who are supposed to protect us. We do not question them because we have enough of a burden just to cope with our own lives. Journalists charged by their profession bring us the truth, too much of the time take the easy way, printing what they are told, rarely looking below the surface. The Watergate exposé is the exception, rather than the rule.

Truth or Money

The media is itself subject to the pressures of the marketplace, which means money. A good example is their attitude toward smoking. They run stories about its deadly effects, they may even ban it in their buildings, but how many newspapers have stopped selling space for tobacco advertisements? Few, if any! Ethically, if they report that smoking is bad, they should be consistent and not sell those ads. Their excuse is that it is legal to advertise smoking products in print (it is illegal on broadcast media like TV). This is a hollow argument, however, because they may refuse to take movie ads for X-rated movies on moral grounds. Is it really more damaging to society to inform people that a theatre is showing an X-rated movie than to promote smoking when tens of unknown thousands of deaths occur per year from smoking? Do you think it could be that they lose little money from the theater's ads, compared to what they get from tobacco companies? Follow the money! The cost of a moral stand is too expensive when it comes to tobacco.

Using Untruths

In dentistry, it is far more lucrative to put in mercury fillings, make crowns, and do root-canals than to not do those procedures. Ironically, one of the ADA's arguments against the anti-mercury dentists is that they are doing it for the money. What a lie! There is no big money in doing plastic fillings. Non-dentists cannot know who is telling the truth unless they follow the money; the highest incomes in dentistry are made by dentists who specialize in root-canals and crowns.

One of the problems for non-dentists is the power of the ADA. They have the ear of the media, they have the power of money for politicians (through their political action committees), and they have the power of licensing laws. The ADA uses all these means and more to quiet those dentists and their allies who are trying to get the truth to the public. The truth will come out eventually, but if the number of sick people who seek out anti-mercury dentists for help is any indication of the extent of the damage, the cover-up is a crime of epic proportions.

Millions of people died unnecessarily in the 1800's from doctor-caused infections, even after doctors were told that the infections were being spread because they were not washing their hands between patients. It took decades before such a simple remedy became common practice. What of the people who died during the delay? Their deaths are just mentioned in passing in the medical history books. What of the doctor who promoted hand washing? He was persecuted and died in an asylum.

There is a lesson to be learned. Unnecessary deaths are still occurring and dentistry is involved. Fortunately, we can correct the problem. We owe it to the victims to be forthright and honest. Mistaken procedures must be eliminated, not covered up. Toxic materials must be removed and people must be helped back to full health. Sweeping the truth under the rug sweeps the victims under the rug, too. We must stop sacrificing people to the ADA's greed and incompetence.

Scientific Studies and Other Lies

The primary source of ill health is poor nutrition. If you get all the nutrients you need, you will have a healthy immune system. If you have a healthy immune system, germs and ordinary toxins cannot harm you. But humans take their natural healing for granted, consistently abusing it with self-inflicted problems from bad habits. Yes, pollution corrupts our environment and the resulting toxins enter our bodies no matter how good our nutrition, but too many of us disregard even what we can control.

So, in our nation of plenty, we have much chronic illness. To treat all this illness, we have what is called a "health care system." Of course, that is not really what it is, but it sounds good. In reality it is an "illness treatment system." Typically, groups in power tend to use words that say the opposite of what is really meant to confuse consumers. An example of one of the new terms being used is "Wellness Center." If you were well, you wouldn't need one!

Media Manipulations

We are constantly told about new studies which support the medical, dental, drug, and food processing industries. Every news program has its medical reporter or even a real doctor to keep the public "informed" of the latest research. It is no coincidence that these reports always seem to favor what these industries believe. Who do you think pays all those scientists who are working so hard to prove that caffeine, nicotine, fluoride, and bungee jumping are safe? Could it be the same people who want you to continue doing business as usual so they can continue making money?

In the 1950's the news shows carried stories showing how DDT could be sprayed around people with no ill effects. News reports showed laughing children enveloped in clouds of DDT spray. Was that for your benefit or the companies promoting the use of DDT? Would you let yourself or your family be enveloped in a cloud of DDT today? Unfortunately, residual DDT is still damaging people in America even though it has been banned for over two decades.

In late 1993 a study was released stating how safe cellular phones are. Who paid for the study? The cellular phone manufacturers! They claimed it was sponsored by the FDA, but FDA officials denied even seeing the study. This is the sort of "research" that robs consumers of their confidence. The new research show that there is reason to fear cellular phones. This new research is being vigorously attacked. In the future, we may look back with horror about how we were duped, just as we do now with DDT.

Scientists For Hire

The way many studies are done, the corporations paying for the study also pay for the conclusion they want. The scientists then make up a study that will give the desired result. If the study comes out against the desired result, the study is redone or the data are falsified. This falsification has been shown repeatedly with nicotine studies sponsored by tobacco companies. The researchers who cannot rationalize their results to the expectations of the group paying for their study find themselves without funds or positions.

High-Level Subterfuge

Recently it was shown that up to a third of all drug studies submitted to the FDA used false data. How then are we to believe a six-year study released in early 1994 showing that certain vitamins are worthless or may even be dangerous for people who have heart disease and lung cancer? This one study contradicts the results of over twenty major pro-vitamin studies published earlier. Would it be too skeptical of us to wonder about the timing of the release of this study--just when the FDA was trying to exert control over the sale of vitamins?

Additionally, there has been scandal after scandal in the scientific journals about other falsified studies. In early 1994 it was found that a doctor had falsified his data in a study on the effectiveness of "lumpectomies" for breast cancer, the study that had brought about a major change in the surgical treatment of breast cancer. The authors of the study said the results are still valid even after the falsified data were removed. If it was your life on the line, would you take their word the second time? Women are justifiably worried about what to believe, as well they should be. Ethical certainty has been reduced to "situational ethics."

Situational Ethics

Our society is being run by situational ethics, which is an outlook that changes "Thou shalt not steal" to "Thou shalt not steal unless you can get away with it!" There are no more absolutes. Individuals decide during each situation what thinks is ethical. A doctor who they would never overcharge patients may think differently if the insurance company is "stupid" enough to pay for extra charges.

This new attitude has changed our ability to trust institutions and individuals that we once took for granted. It is now up to ourselves to find the truth. We must use our brains to decide if we are being used or abused. The basic assumption is that if someone can take advantage of you, they probably are. This assumption may be cynical, but it will be close to the truth.

Call For More Research

When a new idea is promoted that will cause the establishment trouble, the normal reaction is to suppress the idea without appearing to be against it. When mercury came into question, the official response was to "call for more research." The establishment claims to be concerned but has not seen any problems. But, just in case there might be a problem, another study should be funded (by someone else) as soon as possible.

With mercury fillings, the ADA says on one hand that the material has been used for 150 years, so it is "perfectly safe." On the other hand, they suggest that a large, long-term study be done. What they do not acknowledge is that there was concern about mercury since it was first used in 1834. Published studies found fault with using mercury all during those 150 years. Why were these studies not believed? Why have another ten years gone by waiting for another study to be done? Who gains by such a delay? Who loses? You probably already know the answers to those questions.

When a "Dr. Outsider" does a study that is anti-mercury, the ADA does nothing to help it get published. If the ADA wanted to sponsor an "official" study, it would have been done before now. What would happen if the ADA did a study which showed mercury is really as harmful as the anti-mercury believers say it is? They could not suppress the study, ignore it, or ridicule it because it would be their study.

Knowing or Not

In a recent research report it has been shown that people who score low in certain tests think they did much better than they really did. Dr. David Dunning, psychologist at Cornell University, states that most incompetent people do not know they are incompetent. People who do things badly are usually supremely confident of their abilities, even more confident than people who do things well. Their illusion that they know something they do not really know can be source of much trouble. Conversely, those who are the most qualified may actually be less confident in what they do, constantly questioning what they do, and continually seek to improve.

An example of this concept is when you ask an engaged 20-year-old woman about what the first 20 years of her marriage will be like. Her opinions will be absolute and rosy. Ask the same question to a woman who has been married 20 years and her opinions will not be absolute and she may not be able to say anything with certainty.

If this concept is applied to many dentists who think they know what they are doing when they place toxic dental materials or do damaging techniques, they may state with certainty that nothing they are doing will cause their patients any problems. While it is certain in the dentists' mind, it is their patients who will suffer. The truth is that most dentists do not really know what they are doing but only parrot what they were taught in dental school. Their illusion of what is right is just that, an illusion, but the damage they do to patients in their ignorance is real.

When they are challenged by people who really know and understand, they react with hostility. It is beyond their ability or training to understand the reality of their action. They must believe that those who speak against what they do are ignorant. The dentists attack to defend their behavior. Since they are sure they are right, those who oppose them must be wrong. Initially the weight of the numbers of those who do not know seems to sway the outcome.

Truth is hard to bury for long. Truth gains strength with exposure. Slowly others shake off the illusions whether from insight, economic gain or pressure from without. When the fight over toxic dentistry is written about in years hence it will be written as if the ADA saw the dangers and corrected the problems to protect the public. Only those who have fought in the trenches against the ADA's ignorance will know the price that had to be paid.

3

HEARING THE TRUTH

The human mind is like an umbrella –
it functions best when open.

> Walter A. Gropius
> German/American
> architect (1883-1969)

It has been a common experience among all kinds of health professionals that patients do not always act rationally when they are told the truth. They will commonly reject the diagnosis and the doctor who dares tell them, if it is not what they want to hear, rejecting the treatment recommendations along with it. If they are told to quit smoking or drinking or to lose some weight, for example, they are likely to quit listening instead. It is common for patients to not want to hear or discuss a diagnosis of cancer. Family members may be told, but not the patient. People often prefer the illusion to reality, to treat a symptom rather than the cause.

Patients may also leave a doctor who tells them the truth. It does not matter if the doctor showed them a way to overcome the cause of their problem, particularly if the solution involves sacrifice, determination, and discipline. Patients are more likely to follow a doctor who will tell them what they want to hear, whether it is true or not.

Personal Choice

Before you decide whether to clear your mouth of toxic dental materials, think about whether you want to hear the truth or merely vague reassurances. Most people would rather hear that the mercury fillings are "not a problem for most people" than to clean them out to protect themselves from further buildup of toxins. However, if you are going to err, make it on the side of caution. Is it better to have a mouth full of toxic metals and hope you are not affected, or get them out and quit worrying about them?

Plenty of dentists will tell their patients the ADA "line" that mercury fillings are "safe" in most people. Look for a dentist who will guarantee it. If it only affects one in a hundred, ask your dentist to find out if you are that person. He cannot do it. No one can. If the current studies are correct, than it is more like one in five people who are suffering from serious mercury problems. How can these reassuring dentists tell who is affected without a test? Do these dentists do any tests before they place mercury fillings? They do not! You must decide if such vague reassurances, with no guarantees, are enough for you to risk your health.

Be just as cautious of dentists who tell you that they will remove the mercury but only by crowning most of your teeth. They are not offering you the option of a middle ground where you are not being left with toxic metals. You do not have to spend ten thousand dollars to replace them. Use your common sense. Do not be patronized or ripped off. Not only must you be willing to hear the truth, you must sometimes search for it.

Comments by Dr. Harold Loe

Dr. Harold Loe, the recently retired Director of the National Institute of Dental Research, made these observations in a 1993 interview published in *Dental Products Report*:

..Diet plays an important role in controlling high disease (dental caries). Those who have high counts of these organisms (decay causing bacteria) probably have too much sucrose (sugar) in their diet...

We can't settle for just 20 seconds of brushing per day.

That first filling is a critical step in the life of the tooth. Using amalgam [mercury fillings] requires removing a lot of tooth substance, not only diseased tooth substance, but healthy tooth substance as well. [That means mercury should not be used as the first filling!]

Fillings should be as small as possible. Once a large restoration [like a mercury filling] has been placed it cannot be replaced with a smaller one. And, when preparing restorations, AS MUCH HEALTHY TOOTH SUBSTANCE SHOULD BE RETAINED AS POSSIBLE. [Emphasis added]

With the first filling you should do something that can either restore the tooth or retain more healthy tooth substance. Use new materials-composites of materials you can bond to the surface without undercuts.

*So this is a whole new way of practicing
dentistry .. Still, dental schools have
been lagging behind in their teaching. They're still
teaching restorative dentistry as they did 40 years
ago...*
*You have to deal with the disease and then
control the infection. The old concepts are no longer
valid.*

These statements, which reflect the same philosophy as this book, should be the main theme in the *Journal of the American Dental Association* (JADA), not in an article on page 114 of a publication aimed at selling new dental products; maybe one dentist in a hundred even looked at it, maybe only one in a thousand.

If comments are applied to most dental procedures and materials, many, if not most, of the concepts taught in dental school are wrong. The average dentist practicing today graduated 15-20 years ago. The concepts he routinely uses may be much further behind. In fact, much of what is taught has not changed since the turn of the century. The dentistry of 1900 must be given up. It is a hundred years old and as obsolete as a foot-powered dental drill. "Horse and buggy" dentistry must be abandoned.

Those dentists who cannot adapt to the new, more biocompatible, materials should consider retiring. You, as a patient, have the right to demand to be treated in the best way possible. If your dentist cannot use the new materials and techniques in a highly competent manner, do not risk your health as he tries to catch up.

The Busy Dentist

We are all drawn to the concept that "the people who are most busy are the best." Which mechanic is the busiest? Which beautician is the most booked up? Which physician has the fullest waiting room? Which lawyer is the hardest to get to see and the most expensive? It may be true that a high demand for services means those services must be good, but may be the result of many other factors.

An older dentist gave this advice to "help" younger dentists just beginning in practice. He told them that when he first began practice, if he had only two patients scheduled that day, he would schedule them very closely together so they would see each other coming and going and think he was busy. He equated being busy to being successful. But there is a downside to being busy; a dentist can get sloppy about details. When several people are waiting, the tendency is to rush. Who suffers? The dentist suffers excess stress and the patient may get less-than-perfect work. The type of practice you want to find for your own care is one where the office is calm and slow-paced, where the schedule allows five minutes extra, instead of five minutes not enough. If an office is behind schedule, which happens when unforeseen problems arise or the work is more tedious than expected, you should be rescheduled. If the staff does not suggest it, you should. A frazzled, hassled dentist is not who you want doing your fillings.

The In-and-Out Dentist

If your dentist is in and out of the room as he sees one, two or three other patients at the same time, you should be very cautious about having him do your work. If the dentist routinely

57

starts a procedure, then leaves to see another patient, then comes back to do another part of the procedure, then leaves to check another patient, then comes back to finish, while you sit there waiting maybe with your mouth stretched open, you need to find another dentist. Such a dentist will be very distracted and less able to do precise work.

If the dentist is so busy that he turns you over to an assistant to finish the fillings, find another dentist. Composite fillings are considered "technique sensitive," which means they require strict attention to the details or the quality of the filling will be ruined. This procedure takes experience. An assistant will be unlikely to have adequate training and experience to do composite fillings to the degree of perfection required.

Financial pressures may also affect what treatment a dentist chooses. The higher the dentist's overhead, the more crowns he needs to "sell" High overhead is seen in large staffs and a big payroll requires a dentist to really "produce" a lot of high-priced dental procedures.

Personal life style can also force a dentist to "push" crowns. The "big" house, the "big" car and the "country club" life style are all outside forces that may have an influence on what treatments a dentist recommends for you. These are economic forces that patients do not easily discover. The best way to avoid having unnecessary work is to have only basic fillings done.

What Your Dentist Does Not Want You To Know

The information in this book is heresy to most dentists. Heresy is more than just an unorthodox belief; it may also be called unconventional wisdom, meaning ideas that are different than what most people believe. Since arriving at these beliefs did not happen in a day or a month or a year, but over 20 years, it is expected that people with orthodox views will need time to fully consider the truth behind these alternative views. But just because the information in this book is unorthodox does not mean it is not valid.

Dentists will have more reason to react besides the fact that "inside information" has been made public. They may react because this information may cost them money, maybe a lot of money. If a dozen patients in a practice decline having a crown done because they read this book, that is a lot of money.

Dentists may also be angry if you refuse to have a crown done after you read this book because you fear it will cause the death of the tooth and you do not want to have a root-canal done. Crowns and root-canals are big business. Many dentist do only crowns and root-canals. It is no coincidence that dentists who do a lot of crowns also do a lot of root-canals.

Similarly, dentists do not want their patients to question having a cleaning every six months or having X-rays every year. They do not want their patients to ask why they give fluoride treatments to adults or why the health of your gums has more to do with what you eat than how you brush and floss. Their response will be either to dismiss the information in this book as baloney and attack the author or to act as if you dare not challenge them because they are "doctors." You should not tolerate these types of reactions.

Lawyers May Become Involved

Another fear dentists may have is of being sued. The way for dentists to avoid lawsuits is for them to quit doing damage to patients. Perhaps the growing threat of lawsuits is what it will take to get dentists to stop putting mercury in people's mouths.

It has been reported that the largest manufacturer of mercury filling materials in Germany has stopped production because of a change in the German liability laws, holding the manufacturers easily accountable for damage done by the mercury. That is a good example of how public pressure can stop the use of mercury fillings. And if the makers of mercury filling can be held liable, then so could dentists who use this material.

In America the individual dentists are at legal risk although manufacturers have already been sued over the mercury filling materials. Lawyers will not be lenient if the dentist had prior knowledge that mercury is dangerous. Dentists who cite the FDA, which has never approved mercury fillings, and the ADA, which is just a trade organization made up of dentists who use mercury, as authorities in their justification of their use mercury, a well-known poison, will not win the hearts or minds of jurors.

Why Aren't Our Teeth in Better Shape?

If the current methods of treatment were truly helpful, then dental disease would be a thing of the past. It is not! America has more dentists per capita than anywhere else and Americans spend more money on toothpaste, brushes, and floss than any other country. We should all have perfect teeth. Unfortunately, finding a person over 20 without fillings, decay, or gum disease is extremely difficult.

Does it make you wonder what the profession is really about? Maybe it is just a bunch of nice people trying to make a living by helping others but not helping too much so that their "golden goose" will not be killed.

There is more than enough work to do, not because people have unfilled cavities, but because so much damage is being done by well-meaning dentists using toxic dental materials and outdated procedures. It is time for change. The nation is questioning the huge increases in "health care costs" which now account for one-seventh of every dollar spent. Dental work does not account for much of the total, but the effects of dental work may be responsible for much of our illnesses. It is time for dentists to clean up the mess they have made!

4

THE ROLE OF ORGANIZED DENTISTRY

The American Dental Association

The American Dental Association (ADA) is the major "trade" organization for dentists. The Association is powerful nationally, exerting great control through its 50-state organizations and their regional subgroups. The vast majority of dentists are members, and the ADA also has a close relationship with all the dental schools and state dental licensing boards, dominating most of them.

The ADA's attitude toward the mercury "problem" is best expressed as, "What problem?" The organization consistently denies mercury or any other dental material pose any significant problems. Every article published in the *Journal of the American Dental Association* (JADA) claims to be balanced but is always in favor of maintaining the status quo.

Delaying Tactics

What the ADA hopes will happen is that it can ignore the criticism of mercury until a "true substitute" is found. This new material would have to have little or no toxicity, and any dentist would be able to place it with the ease of mercury fillings (this seems to be the ADA's most important criterion). A switch could then happen quietly and the mercury issue would fade away. After a few years were allowed to pass to let the legal "heat" cool down (in other words, letting the statute of limitations for individual suits expire), the ADA could announce how it moved the profession into a new era by getting rid of mercury fillings.

The National Cancer Institute (NCI) recently followed the same pattern regarding diet. The people who believed in a holistic approach to cancer prevention had always stressed anti-cancer diets, which for years the NCI declared as worthless. All of a sudden, the NCT announced that it "discovered" that certain foods have anti-cancer properties. The organization took the credit and went on as if no one else had ever promoted certain foods to be valuable in preventing cancer.

The standard tactic for a large group (that means powerful group) that is being attacked by a vocal minority is first to ignore the attack. If the large group begins to feel threatened, it will attack the speakers, both as individuals and then for their views. If the minority views become accepted by the public or prove to be so overwhelmingly true that further denial is pointless, the large group takes on the minority views as its own and goes on as if it had never been wrong.

However, this process takes a long time to happen, often as long as 50 years, as the leaders who held the original viewpoint are replaced by younger leaders who hold the new viewpoint. This amount of time is reasonable for some kinds of change. If the leaders only wish to "save face," it is understandable as long as NO ONE IS BEING HURT. For example, when the theory of continental drift was first formally proposed in 1920's, it met with strong disapproval, delaying acceptance until the 1970's. No one lost their life or their reputation. But with toxicity from mercury fillings, millions of people are at risk, while dental leaders, who

64

have based their professional careers on the use of mercury fillings, try to "save face."

The ADA knows that if it acknowledges any problem with mercury, attorneys will be lining up to file lawsuits. And if one suit is won, a million more might quickly follow. It is reasonable to believe that attorneys could win against individual dentists since the FDA has never approved the use of mercury fillings, but only approved the ingredients and let the dentists be totally responsible for the mixing and placing of the fillings. Other materials in dentistry are not treated this way.

FDA Works With The ADA

The FDA knows that a mercury filling cannot pass the safety tests it uses for new products. To quell the vocal anti-mercury proponents, it holds meetings, listens to opinions, and then concludes that mercury is "still safe to use" but that "further studies are needed." Many knowledgeable opponents of mercury and other substances that should be banned no longer go to these FDA meetings because they know that the outcome has already been determined before the meetings begin.

The FDA believes that by letting the opposition actually come before its representatives and present their "facts," these opponents will believe that the agency might actually take action. It is no different than a citizen going to a city council meeting and griping. The city council members will nod approvingly at the comments then go ahead and vote the way they had planned to do before the meeting.

Political Reality

People tend to have a simplistic view of how politics work. They believe that telling the truth, showing the facts, and appealing to whomever is in power to "do the right thing," it will sway their opinions and justice will prevail. Lots of luck!

Politics is about power. Those in office have it, you do not. Office holders are beholden to others, who also have power of one kind or another. Their power could come from friendships, relationships, authority, or money. As a result, the truth can become a very small voice in this company. Truth can be rationalized, but a political debt must be paid.

If you were placed on one of these panels of the FDA, who would you listen to first? The FDA, who tells you what it expects the outcome to be, or the group, maybe a university dental school, who sent you as its representative (and who can fire or demote you), or a research center whose future income is dependent on grants from companies who sell the products being denounced? It would be difficult to ignore such pressure.

Imagine you are a delegate to the ADA meeting. You were elected by your friends back home, your golfing buddies or fraternity brothers. Are you going to raise issues that will make you unwelcome when you return home? Are you going to jeopardize your friend's livelihood? Not likely! You will "go along, to get along." It is called the "good old boys club." In our modern society, the professionals are still pressured to conform.

Early Expectations

For years it was expected that the ADA would announce a new position, if not against mercury, at least moving away from its

66

use. If such an announcement had been made in the early 1980's, there would not be such a problem now. Instead, the ADA has taken a "siege mentality," denying all problems and attacking dentists who opposed the organization's position.

In spite of the evidence against it, the ADA continues to strongly support mercury. (Just the risks of birth defects for both patients and the dentist and his staff should be enough to stop its use.) Not only do personal horror stories of the effects of toxic dental materials and treatments abound, but many documented cases exist of healing after proper care. All of these stories and cases are compelling evidence of the mercury problem, but all are ignored as the ADA tries to maintain the status quo.

Millions unknowingly suffer but their plight is ignored. The public may show little mercy for the organization when the tide turns, and turn it will. The end of the ADA may be the public's retribution for the decades of its deceit and denial.

Unfortunately, as it now stands, there is little or no hope that the ADA will come out against mercury or any other toxic material or dental procedure that has been in use for years. The national dental association in Sweden has publicly apologized for its pro-mercury stand now that the country is stopping the use of mercury fillings. Could that happen here? Only if it were the only way for the ADA to stay in existence.

Private Versus Public Positions

The ADA leaders may personally believe that the days of mercury are numbered, but they believe change should happen slowly, that there is no need to cause a panic, that any problems that exist will be dealt with in good time.

However, the individual dentists may not have that luxury. Since these dentists have personally taken the responsibility for whatever they do, they will have to defend themselves. Since they have been informed of the toxicity of mercury, every mercury filling placed after being informed is a potential source of a lawsuit. Each dentist has the possibility of hundreds or even thousands of lawsuits. Anyone who has ever been sued knows that even if you win, the lawsuit can ruin the quality of your life for years. This possibility alone should have made every dentist abandon mercury a decade ago, when, in 1982, the ADA admitted that mercury escapes fillings and enters the body.

If the ADA is not protecting the public, what can you do to protect yourself and your loved ones? The answer is simple: Find someone who knows what they are doing and get your mouth cleaned of toxic metals. If you are sick, then you need to actively work on detoxifying your body.

Second, it is critical to help others who are not as informed as you by taking political action at the grass-roots level and by telling your friends and relatives about your experiences. You could join DAMS (Dental Amalgam Mercury Syndrome), a group made up of people who have been damaged by mercury in their fillings. (See Appendix II.)

Complain on whatever level you can. Some countries, like Japan and Sweden, are working from the environmental damage aspect. (Remember, mercury is declared safe in your mouth, but is considered toxic waste that comes under the jurisdiction of the EPA when it is removed.)

The ADA Position on Research

The ADA says that researching mercury is not its job, stating that it does not do its own research. However, if the organization wanted a study done, it would get it done. If the ADA thought for one moment that a study would show that mercury is safe, it would have been done already. Does the ADA sponsor other studies? Yes. Does it have a research fund? Yes. But the dental material manufacturers and the dental supply companies who contribute funds for research do not want studies done that could be incriminating. To show that the above is true, in December, 1993 a news release reported that a research lab had found an alternative to mercury use. The ADA claimed it had high promise and could be on the market in about three years. However, the news release came from the ADA's Paffenbarger Research Center. Of course, the ADA claims that although mercury is safe, it is developing this new material just in case mercury really does cause all the problems every toxicologist knows it causes. Now what is this amazing new technique? It is a cold welding of tin, silver and gallium with the only thing going for it is its lack of mercury. The assumption is that these metals are neither allergens nor do they cause other immune problems; on the contrary, they do. Another assumption is that these metals do not create electric currents; they do. A third assumption is that these metals do not expand (crack the tooth) or contract (leak); however, they will do one or the other. How easy will these metals be to remove when needing to be replaced? Cold welded metal sounds harder than the mercury fillings. It would be a miracle if this new technique does not cause worse problems than it is supposed to solve.

This new material was called Galloy, and after being tested on adults showed disastrous results. The material deteriorates in the presence of moisture. They must have forgotten about saliva. It was thought that since it breaks down quickly and could not be used for adult fillings, then why not use it in baby teeth? This failed, too. The product was removed from the market quietly in 1998.

The real question is, "Why bother looking for another solution when there are already superior products on the market?" The best answer is composites, which have been available and used for more than two decades. Yet why does the ADA resist recommending their use? After all, the ADA's favorite product researcher, Dr. Gordon Christiansen, has recommended composite over mercury fillings for years. The ADA's reluctance to acknowledge the superiority of composite dental materials over mercury filling materials is beyond logic. The answer to the mercury problem is composites, and they are already here and in use.

The Current ADA View On Composite Fillings

The ADA has been represented in this book as pro-mercury fillings. Its position could also be stated that, although mercury fillings may have "potential" problems, nothing at present exists to take their place. To be sure the reader fully understands the ADA position, an article published in the *Journal of the American Dental Association* in May, 1994, titled, "After Amalgam, What?" by Dr. Karl Leinfelder, a member of the JADA editorial board and Chairman Department of Biomaterials (formerly "dental materials," as the concept of biocompatibility is known in the dental schools) will be reviewed.

His article begins with a short history of the use of mercury in dentistry, summing up that its "greatest incentive" for use was "a relative lack of technique sensitivity." (That means it is easy for dentists to use.) He mentions that the ADA's "stand" is that mercury fillings may be "used without concerns of biocompatibility." This "stand" is why most dentists still use mercury fillings. He admits that the anti-mercury forces may be able to ban the use of mercury in the near future, so alternatives must be considered. First, he refers to some experiments with gallium and tin-based metal fillings before he discusses composite fillings.

He cites research that shows that well-placed composite fillings were still in good condition after ten years. He specifically points out that these fillings were done by "experienced clinicians." His conclusion is that "The problem with posterior (back teeth) composite fillings is more related to the operator than the material." He means most dentists may not be able to do them well because composite fillings are too difficult to do, that is, they are too "technique sensitive." He attributes the early failure of such fillings to dentists making "small mistakes, use of short cuts, and lack of attention to detail." These type of mistakes are common when dentists are rushed because they are trying to see too many patients for composite fillings. Dentists charge more because more time and skill are involved in doing them correctly.

Dr. Leinfelder restates that failure has less to do with the quality of the composite materials than the skill of the dentists when he says the causes for failure of composite fillings "are considerably more related to the operator (dentist) than to the properties of the resin (composite)." He then clearly states the solution when he says that "it is readily possible to avoid these causes of failure by attaining a greater knowledge of the materials used, and the clinical techniques for their insertion." But he seems to believe that dentists cannot improve their skills enough to make the current composite materials usable as replacements for mercury fillings.

He wants the manufacturers to improve the handling characteristics so that composites are as easy to use as amalgam. While this change would be a big bonus because it would lower the costs and shorten the time necessary to remove all the old mercury fillings, it really is an insult to the skill levels of the majority of dentists. He is really saying that dentists should go on using a poisonous material because they are not capable of using a safer material. Furthermore, patients will have to endure the use of mercury, until the manufacturers make composites easy enough for even the most ham-fisted dentist to use. An alternative view that should state if dentists cannot learn to place composites as well as they do mercury fillings, than they should not be practicing dentistry.

The majority of dentists are capable of doing composites well if they can get a fair fee for the service. If mercury fillings are banned, as they will be, dentists will have no alternative but to use composites for most patients. Presently, insurance companies do not adequately reimburse patients who have composite fillings done. For the patients that see things from the viewpoint of lower costs over biocompatibility, this lack of reimbursement puts undue economic pressure on them to choose the cheapest alternative. Dentists who are sensitive to these patients' price complaints feel pressured to place mercury fillings as long as they are legal. These problems will stop once mercury is banned.

The statements in this article about the present quality of the composite materials are refreshingly honest. The true problem seems to lie in the ADA's view of dentists as being too unskilled to use these superior materials. Perhaps it is the ADA's attitude that needs to be improved more than the skills of its members.

Biocompatibility

The question that should be asked before having a filling done is not "How long will the filling last?" but "Is the material biocompatible?" The word "biocompatible" means compatible to life, which, in this case, is your life, a pretty important subject.

You have a right to know about the biocompatability of the treatments you are getting; this right is called "informed consent." (See Appendix I.) The ADA's position is that an Informed Consent form is unnecessary because dental materials are safe. The truth may be that dentists do not want to alarm patients to the potential dangers in their treatments.

Controlling Dentists

Loyalty to a petrified opinion never yet broke
a chain or freed a human soul.
Inscription on bust of Mark Twain in Hall of Fame.

One of the functions of the ADA is to establish a "standard of care" so that it may judge dentists' ability to treat the public competently or better; this is done through uniform educational standards, codes of ethics, and license laws, all proper and reasonable goals. But there can be a negative side to having too much control.

The ADA is not a governing board set up by the public or the government to establish these standards, but rather a trade organization made up of dentists, mainly pro-mercury dentists. These dentists tend to believe that they have all the answers. If a dentist does not fully agree with these standards, this dentist is considered a threat, one who must be controlled to protect the status quo. But since the ADA pro-mercury dentists are currently a majority, they fill most of the positions on the state boards. If the standards are never challenged, they become outdated. More importantly, if the standard is wrong to begin with, maintaining that standard is not in the public interest. Who is to judge whether a standard is right? In dentistry, the standards are judged by the same people who made them.

For example, if a new scientific paper opposes the use of mercury, it will be rejected by every journal supported by groups that believe the use of mercury is a good idea. Then, anyone who searches the scientific journals will find no anti-mercury papers will conclude that there is nothing wrong with using mercury. This is a "Catch-22"!

Only if people are taught to think can they make their own decisions. In dental school, dentists are neither taught to think nor taught to question what they are taught. Instead, they are trained to do dental techniques that comply with ADA concepts. It is critical to train the minds of the dental students to think "like a dentist." (The same training in proper "thinking" goes on in medical schools, law schools, and theological seminaries.) Alternative health practitioners are few because the system of education tries to make all professionals follow the accepted dogma. Challenging even minor concepts is difficult. Although controlling behavior may have some value, if the organization cannot accept more than one viewpoint, it will eventually destroy itself, as all dictatorships do. Before such destruction many people whose interests are supposed to be protected, will be hurt. Dentists are not scientists and most rely on the ADA to tell them what is right and wrong. They believe or follow whatever the ADA says. If they don't believe it, they still follow ADA rules. This scenario sounds more like "mind control" or "behavior control" than leadership. The ADA's position is, "If we cannot convince you to do what we want, we will make your life miserable or revoke your license."

Defining Competence

Are these concepts of "standard of care" and public interest also applied to levels of competence, quality, skill, or even mental impairment? Are quality control standards applied to every dentist? Is any drug test required to determine if a dentist is impaired? The answers are No, No, and No! If the dental lab technicians were to be asked their opinion of the quality of dental work sent to them by dentists, they would tell you it is less than good, sometimes even terrible. Does the ADA check on this? No way! A patient may ask a dentist to remove his mercury fillings and put in composite fillings. If this dentist believes that mercury fillings are bad and recommends that the patient replace them with composite fillings, he is considered to be acting outside the "standard of care." But what if another dentist tells a patient that he should replace his fillings with gold inlays? The ADA would consider that to be a good idea. The ADA says mercury is safe, but if a dentist says it is not, then the dentist is violating the ADA concept of what is "correct." The second dentist may only want to sell some expensive inlays, but that is all right because the ADA claims that gold is stronger and longer-lasting than mercury fillings. Is this duality in the public interest?

National Dental Licensing

Another way the ADA controls dentists is by opposing a national license. The ADA is constantly petitioned by dentists who want to have a national dental license to replace the individual state licenses. Such a change is supported by the vast majority of the ADA membership. As it is now, dentists can only work in the state where they have a license. But the ADA opposes a national license on the basis that it is a "state's rights" issue. The real reason may be that it is much easier to control dentists who must live and work in one area. A dentist who could move anywhere would undermine the ADA control, because they could not be closely monitored.

To dictatorships, too much freedom is a bad thing. Retaining firm control over the individual dentist may be the reason the ADA opposes a national dental license. If it were not the reason, the ADA would go along with the wishes of the members who want to be able to move and still practice dentistry.

Controlling Innovation

Another method to control behavior is to control the pathways of innovation. Typically, the ADA, as most large organizations, tries to maintain the status quo and slow any innovation it finds threatening. Individual dentists who try to respond to the public's desire for safe materials may find

76

themselves in conflict with the ADA's desire to approve any change in the "standard of care" before dentists can use it.

A growing segment of the public is concerned about the environment, both external and internal and do not want mercury in their landfills or their mouths. Can dentists help them or must they refuse because the ADA dogma says mercury is safe?

As of today, dentists cannot oppose the ADA position on mercury without fear of reprisal. The only middle ground is for a dentist to quietly treat patients without using mercury so pro-mercury dentists do not feel threatened.

Source of Change

Attempts to change the ADA's position on mercury have been made since it formed. Only an unscarred optimist would believe that the organization will ever change its position voluntarily. What is the option? Change must to come from the people. Not even the sympathetic dentists can help much. It is a political battle that is up to the people to fight.

The dentists who are believers in using biocompatible dental materials cannot carry the fight themselves. The public must provide support and leadership. Additionally, other interested groups must be recruited. The EPA, environmentalists, sewage treatment professionals, and medical doctors must become involved. As these professionals are shown how these dental materials cause problems outside the mouth, they will find answers to problems they face.

It is sad that the ADA has such power and even worse that the public is being harmed by the organization's abuse of that power. Today, the right to determine what is "correct" lies with people whose interests are power and money, not health. Change can only occur when people reclaim their right to be healthy.

5

HOW THE PRACTICE OF DENTISTRY WORKS

It is not the object of the dental profession to prevent disease but to fix it after it happens. The way payments are made is that the most money goes for the most manipulative treatments; root-canals, crowns and implants. Is any money paid to help balance your body chemistry so you will not need treatments later? Not a penny. On the contrary, dentists who tried to provide such services were attacked and had their licenses suspended. If dentists try to do it right and end up not being paid and risking their livelihood, they learn quickly to change back to the drill, fill, and bill attitude. Of course, these procedures are small potatoes. Now dentists want to "prep, crown, and retire."

It is a common complaint in our office that it seems expensive to get all the dental junk out of their mouths. It may seem expensive because it must be paid for out of their pocket and all at once. I had a kidney stone removed in a hospital for which the insurance paid $10,000. I got rid of the next kidney stone with five dollars worth of herbs. I had to pay for the herbs out of my pocket. To clean up the dental mess in your mouth and spend $3000 out of pocket is better than if you have the insurance pay $50,000 in medical bills.

It is common for patients with chronic sinus problems to have had sinus surgery, often more than once, as well as years of suffering. All those bills are covered by insurance. If their problem comes from a root-canal and the sinus problem stops when the tooth is extracted, it may not be covered. The cost of breast cancer surgery and reconstruction is covered but removing the root-canals on the breast meridian may not be.

After WWII wages were frozen. Adding a pre-tax benefit of health insurance was a way to offer more money without violating the law. By not paying income tax on the health insurance benefit seemed like a great idea to everyone. The result was the mental attitude that we were getting something for nothing. What really happened was we quickly lost the ability to know the cost before the services are performed. Hospitals and physicians were able to set up a direct payment of whatever they want without our ability to say anything.

Huge medical costs have now numbed us. Many older Americans can remember when a hospital room cost $50 a day. When it hit $100 it was shocking. Now they do not charge a flat rate for the room but line-item everything. Forty-dollar disposable pillows and five-dollar aspirins are the norm. If you have to pay for medical services out of pocket, the price would drop like a stone. The new medical accounts may help bring things into balance. It is the money driving the system and the insurance trap means they have access to it and you do not have any say in the matter.

Many people will get upset if they have to pay up to $5000 to completely redo their dental work but never think twice about driving their new SUV out of the showroom and losing the same amount of money; this is an attitude. If you want to get well, you have to face it and get through it. Make a long-term loan to minimize the impact but realize that there is only one way to do it and that is to get it done.

While it does cost to have fillings replaced, do not let anyone talk you into crowning teeth to do it. If there is a mercury filling, it should be possible to replace the filling with another filling. Many people wanting to get their mercury out are manipulated into crowning their teeth. The expense can be so great that they can only do half of their teeth. Now they have half of their mouth with crowns and the other with mercury fillings. That is not sane. Do not let this be done to you. First, get the metal out, the root-canals out, the crowns out. One possibility is to put temporary crowns on so that all of the metal is out. Then go back and replace the temporaries later (within a year). Do not end up half and half.

A sobering realization came to me when patients who moved away and then returned with several new crowns in their mouths. The warnings to the patients were not sufficient as the new dentist just looks at their teeth and tells them they need a couple of crowns. Why not do it since they have insurance? Knowing they did not have any need when they left and they did not break any teeth, it is obvious they were a victim of the push for crowns so common in most dental practices.

Dentists are encouraged to crown teeth. They are told that new patients are where the big money is. Dentists are given statistics as to what is the current value to their practice of new patients. Dentists are told they need to get as many new patients as possible. Special courses to teach dentists how to do examinations and "case presentations."

A case presentation is what happens when patients are told by a dentist the condition of their teeth, gums and bone, and how he plans to fix (restore) it, and how you can pay for it. The interesting thing is many or even most patients do not follow the dentists' recommendations. Five years later they often still do not have any problems with what is already there. It is a buyer beware situation.

New Dentist

When new dentists set up their offices, they usually buy the latest equipment, using this "hi-tech" as a patient draw showing that they are on the cutting edge; this helps cover up their lack of experience. It probably takes years, maybe ten years to get their skills near their maximum. Dentists in their forties and fifties are considered at their peak. Many dentists do not change any of their techniques after this period but are focusing on building enough money to retire. Buying the latest equipment is not feasible for older dentists as there are too few years left to pay it off. With the new equipment, like lasers, digital X-rays, and air abrasion costing so much, it would take a decade to re-equip their offices. That idea does not take into account the extra training and changes in their practice. This does not mean dentists in their twenties, thirties, and sixties are not good dentists, but it does mean you must be that much more careful.

"You're The Doc"

"You're the Doc" is a common expression by patients. It is nice that people have faith in professional but not blind faith. Everything a professional tells you should be analyzed to make sure it is what you want, that you think over the consequences and accept the results. It would be nice to believe every professional makes every decision correctly and in their patients' best interest.

Other forces drive professional decisions; money, energy, convenience, sobriety, and insurance. For instance, is the drug recommended the best one or did a good-looking drug rep just take the doctor out to lunch where the virtues of the newest drug were explained, as well as a bonus plan where the doctor receives perks if they prescribe the drug? Or did the dentist just return from a seminar where he was admonished for not doing 20 crowns per week? There are many other possibilities that you could imagine. Every one you can think of has already occurred somewhere to someone. Many doctors have substance abuse problems, divorce problems, "keeping up with the Jones" problems, college tuition payments, and the worst one, wrong training.

Doctors may make the best recommendation they are capable of making and they still could not be in their patients' best interest. It is important that you do not fall victim to thinking that the doctor always knows best. You must use your own brain. A minor illustration: A patient had all his mercury fillings removed, needed a new filling and told the dentist to put in a white filling and the dentist said he would. After the decay was removed, the dentist told the patient that the cavity was too large for a white filling and he had to put in a mercury filling. The patient quietly agreed.

When he came to our office to have it replaced, it turned out to be a rather small filling with no difficulties whatever. It seemed the dentist probably never planned to do the white filling. The patient should have told him that the agreement was to use a white filling and if the dentist did not feel capable of completing it, he should place a temporary. The patient would not pay for it either, since the service was not done as agreed. It does require a certain amount of assertive behavior that we have all been trained not to do out of politeness or respect. It is your body and you do not have to let anyone put toxic materials into it and pay for the privilege.

Another example is heart bypass surgery. We have all heard of patients who have gone into the hospital for tests only and the doctors admit them and do open heart surgery the next day. They tell patients that they cannot let them go home, as they could die that very night. They make their case in such a way that patients are happy they got to them in time and saved their lives. Sounds good but it is not true. While you might die during the night they let you go home, the odds are against it. The odds are greater that you will die on the operating table during the five-hour operation. After all, the patient was so sick they might die, but are healthy enough to go through a traumatic surgery. If the patient had no insurance or any way to pay a non-bypass option would suddenly be found

Types of Dental Practices

The way dentistry is practiced is changing. Originally, all dental practices were fee-for-services except for government clinics. Now there are many kinds. The types of practices are Fee-for-service, Preferred Provider Organization (PPO's) and Dental Maintenance Organizations (DMO's), capitation, retail, and insurance. Most offices will be a mix of several payment types with different fees for each group. Some may get lower fees for less service. Others will get lower fees and the same service with full-fee patients subsidizing the lower fee patient. (That is what happens at hospitals now.)

The traditional fee-for-service office will become the smallest part of the whole profession in the near future. Fee-for-service offices will be made up of dentists who do the most elaborate work, cosmetic services, and holistic dentists. They may take insurance assignment but more often nowadays they expect cash payments and the patient gets the reimbursement checks.

PPO's and DMO's are the insurance companies' attempt to push dentistry into the medical mold. These programs have not grown much, as dentists have strongly resisted the financial pressure put on them. They negotiate a lower fee with the dentists who sign up, so the insurance companies can offer lower costs to the companies. Some fee-for-service offices take some PPO patients, particularly if they are not busy. If a patient does not go to a dentist on their list, the amount paid drops. This system is a powerful way to control people.

Capitation dental offices work only on patients who have a negotiated contract. A union might make a deal with certain dental offices so they will do procedures at a reduced fee, but in return the dentist gets all the union members and their families as patients.

The largest group is those patients covered by dental insurance. This group has grown from zero in 1960 to 40 percent of patients today. These patients get a pre-tax payment deduction the same as medical insurance model. This group may have peaked, as insurance companies try other methods to offer lower premiums to the companies.

There is a growing retail dentistry with storefront offices staffed by dentists who are not committed to the practice but to their take-home pay. Each time you go in you may be seeing a different dentist. To those patients who believe one dentist is the same as another, this does not seem to be a problem because they do that at their physician's office now. These retail offices offer expanded hours, evenings and weekends which is a convenience that attracts a lot of customers, but not biocompatibility.

Retail practice may be attractive because many dentists welcome getting out from under the business side of the dental practice. They become an employee with regular benefits. This type of practice is particularly attractive to the growing number of female dentists who can more easily balance raising a family and work. Such a practice can be attractive to all dentists who see it as a way to make more money by doing more per hour, maximizing efficiency and by using trained auxiliaries. There may be an emphasis on selling crowns if the dentist is paid on commission.

Retail dentistry, PPO's, and DMO's are not conducive to holistic dentistry, which is time-consuming. People who are sick require even more time as they can handle less treatment at a time and are more sensitive to materials and techniques used. Do not expect these practices to change the way they practice to accommodate you.

It is only common sense to prevent people from getting sick. If earlier dental treatment was the cause of the illness, then doing more of the same will not help. A spiral of declining health may result that is more expensive to reverse, if it can be reversed. Many people who are ill from dental techniques or materials have had the quality of their lives lowered to the point that it requires all their energy just to get through the day. Even if you do have some type of insurance coverage, it may be better to forget about it than to let it decide your future health. You must decide if you want to trade your health to save an insurance company money or make life easier for the dentists.

Insurance

Economics drives the system and the more insurance companies are involved, the more the bottom line will control what is done. Insurance companies are not the least interested in whether a material is toxic, believing that is the dentist's choice. They are only bothered when attorneys get involved. It is economics, not biocompatibility, that drives the system.

Biocompatibility was poorly understood when mercury was introduced but even then, many were against its use. Ignorance of natural law can exact a terrible price. Being ignorant of the law of gravity does not mean you will not fall down. Ignorance of toxic materials does not protect you from being poisoned. Thorium was used for fillings around the time of the Civil War. No one knew it was radioactive because radioactivity was not discovered until later. The people who had the thorium fillings paid with shortened lives. Such life-shortening practices are still going on despite modern knowledge of materials' effects.

As an individual, you have to decide if you are going to control what is done to you or are going to allow a line in an insurance contract determine your fate. We hear a constant complaint on the news that an insurance company will not pay for this or that procedure. It is a phony argument made to keep people confused and lawyers busy.

Insurance will pay for whatever is negotiated in the contract. If a cost is in the contract and prepaid, they will cover it, although reluctantly. If they do not pay for something they should cover and they are not called on it, they get to keep the money. If a procedure is not in the contract, then they will not cover it nor should they. If your policy says it does not cover braces then it matters not if they are needed; it is not a gray area.

Insurance policies are written so the insurance companies are only responsible for the least expensive procedure that can be done. When it comes to fillings, the insurance companies will pay for the cheaper mercury fillings rather than the more expensive white fillings. With insurance companies you get what you pay for minus their 20 percent fee to handle the paper work.

Actually, dental insurance is not insurance. Insurance is needed when your house gets destroyed by a tornado, an unlikely event. Having dental checkups twice a year is not a risk but a predictable event. Dental insurance is really prepaid dental benefits. You pay for them directly or indirectly plus the premium the insurance company takes for their trouble.

Real insurance covers most or all of the costs of a tragedy. Dental insurance has a low upper limit per year of approximately $1000 to $1500. If you are trying to have your work all done in a year, you will not get more than the maximum listed on the contract. Spreading the costs out over several years is not in the patient's best interests but does favors the insurance companies. If your house was destroyed by a tornado, the insurance company would not say, "We will pay you $1500 this year, but you must wait until next year for another payment." This further illustrates that dental insurance is not really insurance.

Medical Costs

We all know that plastic surgery is expensive and not covered by insurance. Then why is it being done more and more? Because that is what the people who buy it want. It seems to matter not that many plastic surgeons make more than a thousand dollars per hour and heart surgeons make ten thousand dollars per operation and may do more than one per day. That sounds good but there are new treatments that make these doctors seem underpaid. A new tonsillectomy costs two thousand and takes less than five minutes and that includes the doctor explaining the procedure.

The most lucrative treatments are the new laser eye surgery. It takes five to ten minutes and costs $4000 uninsured. People are moved through the laser surgery at six to ten per hour. Twenty-five patients gross a hundred thousand dollars per day. And people are lining up for the surgery.

The usual patients in our office wait in dread for the estimate. They exclaim, "I don't have insurance" as if most other people have someone footing their dental bills. This idea that insurance covers people's medical and dental expenses is a con job fostered by those in government who want people to be dependent on the government. Someone is paying for those medical bills and they are taking out a nice percentage for their trouble. People forget how much is taken from their pay, anted up by their companies (in lieu of a raise) or paid by taking money from people making more money. Hospitals overcharge (legally required by federal law) to cover people who do not have insurance or just do not pay.

Patients will gladly suffer the most awful treatments because they are covered. They will have open-heart surgery rather than chelation (chemical bonding to remove metal) treatments. Patients undergo chemotherapy, when studies show it is not effective, because it is covered. They will wear glasses all their lives since they are covered and the laser surgery is not. The list is endless. Persons who have found the effectiveness of alternative medicine know countless examples. People who have given up on the medical system or who have been given up by the medical system may have not learned this yet but soon will.

We have been brainwashed into believing that the U.S. medical system is the world's best. We know if we think about it that this could not be true or we would not be so sick. How can we be healthy if every other ad on TV is for an over-the-counter remedy or a new ad for prescription drugs? America ranks far down on the list in overall health compared to the other industrialized nations, while we spend more than any other country.

One-seventh of every dollar spent in America goes toward "healthcare." [The highest in the world.] It was not long ago it was one dollar in ten. How much do we have to spend to be healthy? We could spend every dollar and it would not be enough when the real cause of sickness is found within the health care system. It is well-known that the people who die by medical mistakes exceed all the other causes of death, except illness, more than car accidents, gun deaths, accidental deaths combined.

Dentists are right in the middle of this tragic treatment, as we use every toxic metal we can find. We treat the mouth, as it is not part of the body. Dentists think that what they do to the mouth has no impact on the rest of the body. The lack of knowledge about the effects of dentistry on the body adds greatly to the sickness in our country. It is not improving and may well get worse in the next 20 years. There is only one way to protect yourself and that is by taking control over what any health professional does to you. You have to be educated and assertive to protect yourself. If you are not in control of your own health, you will be controlled by someone else.

Managed Care

The buzzword in medicine during the 1990's was "managed care." Patients do not want managed care; they want cures. The difference between managing a disease and curing it is where the big money is. If you cure someone, the income stream of dollars stops, but if you manage their disease, you can collect for the rest of their lives.

Can you name any diseases that have been cured? Probably none but smallpox. How about diseases that are just managed and not cured?--heart disease, diabetes, HIV, MS, kidney disease--and the list goes on and on. Constant charity money drives tell you the cure is just around the corner. Actually, cures are not being sought, only ways to manage the illness, allowing the patient to at least partially function, while the money keeps flowing in. It might seem a bit cynical but history proves it out. Life spans are another one of the ways we are misled about how healthy we are. At the turn of the century the death rate among children was as high as one in four. My father had seven siblings and lost two. I had three siblings and lost one. Such deaths are much less common now but we only owe some of that to our health care system, mainly antibiotics. The fewer number of deaths was due to improvements in the water supply, sewage systems and better nutrition (until recently).

To tell if the life span for the rest of us is better, you only have to compare the statistics of the population of adults 100 years ago and those of today. Without the early deaths of children factored in, the life span has only increased a few years, not the 30 years the media keeps telling us. Here are some examples from the standard reference book by Bogue. To show how the statistics are distorted by childhood disease, here are a few numbers. A one-year-old in 1900 has a life expectancy of 49 years. A one-year-old in 1995 has a life expectancy of 75 years or 26 years more. Once they survive childhood the difference drops dramatically. A 20-year-old in 1900 has a life expectancy of 63 years. Just surviving childhood added 14 years. By contrast, a 20-year-old in 1995 only adds 2 years to 77. By the time a person reached 70, the difference was just a few years and not the 26 years statistics try to make us believe.

We are constantly told that the life span in 1900 was about 50 years. If that were true than where did all the old people come from? Old people lived throughout recorded history. Many of the fathers of our country lived long lives: Franklin lived 84 years, Jefferson 83, Adams 91, Washington 67 and he died after they bled a gallon of blood out of him. So how can they think we will believe people died at 50 years of age? They think we are gullible and will believe any statistics they tell us, and they might be right.

The media make a big deal out of people living to be 100. How many do you know? Probably not many, because the odds are 1.4 per 10,000. During one TV show in January 2000, where they discussed the coming 100 years, it was predicted that one person in 100 would reach 100 years of age by the end of the next hundred years. That number should not give many people comfort, when so many are dying before they are seventy or even fifty.

The reason any of these people reach 100 either now or ever is good genes and luck. Healthy living is only a small part of it. Most of us have to do the best we can with the maverick genes we inherited. Do not be led astray by misapplied statistics. The length of your life is not determined by statistics. We must focus more on preventing premature deaths and lives of crippling, degenerative diseases.

Another possibility is that the predictions may all be wrong. Life spans may not be getting longer and may begin dropping as some have predicted. Older Americans (more than 70 years of age) were raised before the processed foods took over the marketplace after WWII. Kids now are raised on fast foods. The bodies built with processed foods will not be nearly as healthy as those built on the whole foods eaten in the first half of the 20th century. Watch the obituaries and see how many people are dying in their forties, fifties, and sixties.

While we are outspending the world on health (sickness) care, we see our diabetes rate skyrocketing. Rates of other diseases are getting worse, too. Asthma, many cancers, Parkinson's, Alzheimer's, multiple sclerosis (MS) and amytrophic lateral sclerosis (ALS), to name a few. And it is not just that more people are getting these diseases but that they are getting them at a younger and younger age.

How can we be as healthy, as they say, and still be so sick? Why do we need to spend a seventh of our national income on medical care if we are so healthy? Something is wrong, and we need to stop believing the razzle-dazzle and see the truth. It is the baby boomer generation that is taking the first hit of ruined health. Their children and grandchildren will be worse. All the B.S. about genetic therapy is not going to be the answer. Our bodies are the same as those of the caveman. We must follow the needs of our bodies or suffer the consequences. We ignore this basic truth and pay with chronic illness and a shortened life.

We are being used to feed the medical money machine, but can choose to live another way. We can take better care of ourselves and resist being swept into the insurance trap. The way that trap sucks you in is that if you do what the medical monster wants, you get insurance coverage. If you opt for alternative treatments, you must pay for it yourself--pure economics.

Drugs

The money spent on drugs is staggering. The monthly bill for drugs for a heart transplant patient is $2500. The new monthly shot for MS (that has mixed results) is $1000 each. AIDS patients can take up to 100 pills in a single day. Each new drug is many times as expensive as the earlier ones and each one has side effects that often require additional drugs to control. We burden the elderly with so many prescriptions; they spend all their time keeping track of their pills. We see that Americans are charged two to four times the price our neighboring countries pay for the same drugs from the same manufacturers. Have you noticed all the giant new pharmacies being built all across our country? Follow the money.

The answer is not lowering our costs by trying to get the federal government to pay for drugs. It is most important to know that the drugs we take actually do little good; most just alter symptoms while causing more problems. People must learn what they are taking, why, and what the side effects are. If you cannot answer these questions, it is time to do your homework. To underscore the seriousness of the problem with drugs, it has been reported that as many as one-fourth of all drug studies have doctored data so they look better than they actually were. In the February, 2000 edition of the *New England Journal of Medicine*, the editor apologized because he had found 19 instances in three years where positive results were reported in

94

their journal where researchers had a financial interest in the outcome of a study.

The research for new drugs is so expensive that what really happens is that when a new drug is released, data is collected to see what really happens. The public is used as the guinea pigs. If too many report adverse side effects, as with the sleeping pill, thalidomide, the drug may be removed from the market. It took 47 deaths to stop the marketing of one arthritis drug. You must be careful when taking any new drug. Do not think the doctor is being kind in giving you samples he happens to have for you to try. Beware!

In other countries there is not an operating team sitting around waiting for a possible patient as there is in America. Study after study shows that heart patients can be well managed by a cardiologist using other treatments including drugs. Is there any reason you could think of why the doctors might not want people to go home and think about it? What do you think would happen if the patient responded to the call for instant surgery with, "I'd love to get this done tomorrow. I don't have any insurance and I'm sure I could pay you once I get back on my feet." Do you think that the doctors would find many ways that the patient could get along without the surgery?

While dentists are not quite as efficient as the heart surgeons, they do have ways of encouraging patients to comply with their treatment recommendations. Numberless courses are offered to teach dentists the verbal techniques and financial methods to get patients to "accept the best dentistry has to offer." That term usually means crowns but has expanded into cosmetic dentistry and implants.

Dentists are told that there is a million dollars of undone dentistry in their patient files. They are told that only half of the patients follow their recommendations. You must wonder if all the people who decline the recommended treatment have had their teeth fall apart. Patients in our practice that declined crowns we recommended decades ago, when we did as other dentists do, seem to still be getting along fine. Every dentist who has been in practice more than 10 years has seen the same thing. We suggest the same old rule, "Let the Buyer Beware."

6

MERCURY IN YOUR MOUTH

Mercury Fillings

In 1845 the dentists of the American Society of Dental Surgeons said, "...the use of all amalgams (mercury filling materials) is malpractice."

When people think of fillings, they generally think of mercury fillings, the standard fillings used by most dentists for back teeth and in front teeth where they cannot be seen; they are the fillings that look black or grey.

These fillings are commonly called by two other names. The name many dentists like is "silver fillings," which is not as accurate because silver only makes up 25-30 percent of the filling, while mercury comprises 50 percent. When dentists first began to use fillings, the only choice was gold. By using the term "silver filling," the patient still must have felt they were getting a filling that had monetary value, just as silver money had value. The most common term used by dentists is "amalgam." The definition of amalgam is a "metal alloy of mercury." This term is not really accurate either because mercury fillings are not true alloys of mercury. The mercury does not combine molecularly with the other metals (tin, zinc, and silver). As with the term "silver fillings," the use of the term "amalgam" hides the fact that fillings are made with mercury. The public is not familiar with most of the metals in the fillings or metallurgical terms, but they do know mercury is

97

poisonous. The most accurate and least deceptive term is "mercury fillings;" thus, it will be the term used throughout this book.

Since much of the mercury in fillings is "free-mercury," not bound to any other metal, it can vaporize, leave the filling, and enter the body. This can happen any time, but much more is released during and after chewing. The mercury escapes as mercury vapor, which is then inhaled. Almost 100 percent of the inhaled mercury vapor is absorbed instantly through the lungs or nasal passages. The mercury absorbed in the nasal passages can enter the brain directly. The mercury absorbed through the lungs goes into the blood, which goes directly to the heart, and from there is sent throughout the body. The mercury does not stay in the blood because it is so actively adsorbed, or absorbed by the cells of the body, meaning it either stays on the cell membrane's outer layer or enters the cell.

The presence of mercury in the body is bad, because mercury is one of the most toxic of all metals, poisoning every cell it enters, particularly attracted to the nerve cells, including the brain. Mercury has a long list of side effects, including birth defects; once absorbed, it is very difficult for the body to remove.

Since everything in the above paragraph is true, why is there a controversy about whether mercury should be banned? Is it to protect dentists from liability? How is it possible that the federal government, including the Food and Drug Administration (FDA), knows the facts but still allows this poison to be used in over 150 MILLION American citizens?

It is noteworthy that any mercury filling material left after a tooth is filled is considered toxic waste and must be disposed of, according to guidelines established by the Environmental Protection Agency (EPA). It is also noteworthy that putting mercury filling material into a landfill is against the law. If it can poison a landfill, how can it be safe in your mouth? Are people so blindly obedient to authority that they cannot see through the lies and half-truths that are used to defend the indefensible?

Most people remember the fairy tale, "The Emperor's New Clothes," in which everyone believed what they were told because they were afraid to admit the truth, which was right before their eyes. It took a child, who had not yet learned to doubt the truth which he could see with his own two eyes, to tell the simple truth. It is the same with mercury fillings. One merely has to look at the facts to exclaim the truth, MERCURY IS POISONOUS AND SHOULD NOT BE USED IN THE HUMAN BODY. There it is. All the denial in the world cannot change that fact.

Why would anyone want a poisonous metal in their body, when no one knows how much of it a person can tolerate before becoming ill? The question should be, "Why should anyone tolerate it when there are much safer alternatives available?" No good can come from contaminating your body with mercury. No quality of life is made better. There is no biological need for mercury, and it can only damage your body's biological functions. Therefore, the use of mercury in dentistry is a violation of the public trust and should be banned immediately.

Furthermore, no amount of protest from dentists and their organizations should stop the ban. If they could prove mercury is safe, they would have done it years ago. Lies, evasions, and half-truths are all the public hears from them. It is time to quit listening to the lies and follow the obvious truth. As the child in the fairy tale said, "Look everyone, the Emperor isn't wearing any clothes!

Evading The Truth

A half truth is a whole lie.
Yiddish proverb

Every lie and half-truth the American Dental Association (ADA) has used to defend mercury has been answered with the truth by many anti-mercury dentists. But it is not the anti-mercury dentists who should have to show it is dangerous; it is the doctors using mercury who must show proof of its safety. To play their word games is to delay banning mercury in fillings, which should have been done decades ago. If the mercury-using dentists can continue their delaying tactics, it may be another 20 years before the mercury materials are removed from the dental offices. How many more lives will be ruined by this poison for each year of delay?

The poisonous effects of chronically inhaling mercury from fillings are well known by the ADA and the federal government. Every product sold in America must have a Material Safety Data Sheet (MSDS) which describes the product's physical properties, health problems, fire risk data, and other hazards associated with it. The MSDS on the mercury sold to dentists by dental supply companies specifically states what damage can result from exposure to mercury. The list of health hazards on the MSDS used by most of the companies who sell mercury states:

"Chronic (long-term exposure): Inhalation (breathing it in, as from fillings) of mercury vapors causes mercurialism. Findings are extremely variable and include tremors (shakes), salivation (excess saliva), stomatitis (inflammation of the

*mouth), loosening of the teeth, blue lines on the gums (tattoos), pain and numbness in the extremities (multiple sclerosis symptoms), nephritis (inflammation of the kidney), diarrhea, anxiety, headache, weight loss, anorexia, mental depression, insomnia (sleeplessness), irritability, instability, hallucinations, and evidence of mental deterioration (Alzheimer-like symptoms)." ***
(From MSDS, issued by the Caulk Dental Company.)

That list does not make mercury sound like a safe material to use. Just think how common some of those symptoms are in our country. Anxiety, headache, and depression are common! Kidney disease is a leading cause of death. Many of these symptoms cause a severe loss in the quality of life.

Has your dentist read the MSDS sheet on mercury? He might have, but do not count on it. The dentist cannot say that he has not had a chance to see the MSDS because he is required by law to have MSDS's for every product he uses on file in his office. The dentist may have been "too busy" for the past few years to read it, but do not let someone hurt you and yours through disinterest and ignorance. It is your responsibility to protect yourself and your family.

Amalgam (Mercury) Tattoos

There is some confusion about amalgam or mercury tattoos. They are just like a tattoo on your skin that is made by forcing metal-containing inks under the skin to leave a mark. Amalgam tattoos appear dark blue to black depending on how much mercury is present. They can be tiny to huge.

There are several ways that these tattoos can be formed. They can be the result of galvanic (electric) current where mercury comes out of the filling and deposits into the tissue next to the tooth. They can be due to the gums being damaged during the removal of an old filling or during crown preparations. (It is common to see a blue ring around a crowned tooth.) Tattoos are often seen after an apicoectomy where the end of the cut root is sealed with a mercury filling. These can be very deep into the bone and large depending how sloppy the dentist was during the placement.

Some times actual pieces of mercury fillings will be left in the gums or in the bone. If a tooth is extracted the same day a mercury filling is done or replaced, a scrap of mercury filling material can easily fall into the open socket. (If a rubber dam is used there would be a much reduced chance for this to happen.)

With either a tattoo or an actual piece of mercury left in the gums or bone, there is an attempt by the body to remove it one molecule at a time. Unfortunately, it will take more than a lifetime for your body to remove such a large concentration. The only way to get rid of tattoos or pieces left is to physically remove them. This can usually be done by removing a piece of gum tissue using several different techniques or when it is in the bone by removing bone around it.

It is common to find multiple tiny spots of mercury hidden within the gums during gum surgery. There is also a high concentration of mercury within gum tissue next to a mercury filling even without a visible tattoo. This toxic gum tissue looks normal to dentists because dentists are used to seeing swollen and red tissue around fillings because mercury causes this inflammation. Inflamed gum tissue may be normal in our country but it is not healthy. It is easy to remove this toxic tissue when the teeth are extracted but it is not routinely done. It is never removed when fillings are just replaced but it may be worth some research to see if gum tissue should be routinely removed when the mercury fillings are removed.

If dentists do not think mercury fillings are dangerous then they will not consider mercury tattoos to be a problem. When you have your fillings replaced, you need to ask if you have any tattoos and ask that they be removed. It would be prudent to ask that swollen gum tissue next to the filling be removed, too. It makes no sense to get the fillings out and leave mercury in the gums.

ADA Admits Mercury Escapes Fillings

Over 20 years ago the ADA admitted, reluctantly, that it knew that mercury is released from mercury fillings. Up to that point, the organization had officially denied the truth, even though it was known to the scientific community since the 1930's and maybe even earlier. The truth had been suppressed for at least 50 years. After the ADA admitted to lying about mercury being released, many dentists thought that mercury would be banned immediately. Instead, the ADA proposed a new lie: "Although mercury does come out of the fillings, the amount is so small that it cannot hurt you." Even with its history of misinformation, dentists accepted this new lie and it is still the "official" ADA line.

The ADA was probably surprised that after admitting it had lied before, anyone would believe this new lie. Americans, being basically honest, trusting people, believe that professional groups are basically honest, too. They forget that the whole purpose of such groups is to further their own viewpoints and strengthen their control over their areas of interests. When your best interest collides with their self-interest, which do you think wins? They follow what is best for themselves, which is to be expected of any group no matter how lofty their goals.

Unfortunately, most Americans believe that their government agencies, and groups such as the ADA, will protect them all the time and in all matters. People may believe the famous line, "Hi, I'm from the government and I'm here to help you." The truth is the government protects its own interests above yours. For example, until recently, Congress routinely passed laws that you must obey, while exempting themselves and other government officials from having to obey the same laws.

The Public Believes ADA

The ADA seems to believe that people believe everything it says, no matter if it is truth, half-truth or an outright lie. Up until now, it seems that the ADA is right because people are taking its word on many important matters and are not challenging its veracity. The ADA also seems to have tremendous power with the media. The organization has used its clout to obscure the truth and the media has believed it. Even the TV news magazine program, "60 Minutes," was subjected to tremendous pressure after it brought the message of mercury toxicity to national television in December of 1990. Even though this was one of the show's most popular segments, there was no follow-up or even a rebroadcast during its summer reruns.

If people dropped dead immediately after a mercury filling was placed, the ADA would probably still deny any connection. Is it any wonder that because the effects only develop after years of accumulation of mercury in the body that the ADA denies any association? There is enough mercury in one average filling to kill someone, if the person's body absorbed it all at once; that should be proof enough of mercury's toxicity.

If Mercury Fillings Were Just Being Introduced

When looked at objectively, composites are approaching perfection compared to the sorry materials of the past. If the only materials available were composites, and someone tried to introduce mercury fillings, they would be run out of town. Imagine you are at your dentist's office and he says, "You need a composite filling that will cost a hundred dollars, but if you want, we have a new material made using a fifty-percent concentration of toxic mercury, that we can use and it will only cost sixty dollars." Would you say, "Go ahead, Doc, give me the cheaper toxic stuff"?

In addition, if mercury filling material were just being introduced, the EPA, OSHA and the FDA would all be adamant against its use. Dental employees would quit their jobs because of the dangers in handling mercury. The groups fighting birth defects would picket.

Mercury Causes Birth Defects

The chemicals we ingest may affect more than our own health. They affect the health and vitality of future generations. The danger is that many of these chemicals may not harm us, but will later do silent violence to our children.

Senator Abraham
Ribicoff, 1971

The fact that mercury causes birth defects should also be enough to ban it. The number of birth defects has increased 500 percent since 1940 and is as high as 15 percent of all births. One would think that the March of Dimes would fight to ban the use of all mercury. This is an outrageous burden for individuals as well as for our society to bear just to continue to use toxic dental materials. (The book *Infertility & Birth Defects* by Sam Ziff and Michael Ziff, D.D.S. discusses these problems and their link to mercury.)

The fact that mercury attacks the nervous system should make the people with multiple sclerosis (MS) take it seriously because the symptoms are the same. The damage of Alzheimer's disease could also be caused or aggravated by mercury, as shown in recent studies. The national societies that were formed to help find solutions to these illnesses should be concerned about any connection with mercury fillings and should not be reassured by the ADA and FDA statements that mercury fillings are not to blame.

Other Health Problems

Most people are aware that mental depression is a problem in America. Estimates of up to one-third of all Americans suffer from depression sometime during their life. Millions are suffering depression at this moment. These people are treated with billions of dollars of medical care.

It would seem reasonable to remove their mercury fillings before placing them on a lifetime of antidepressant medicine that has many serious side effects.

Do you know anyone with kidney problems? Kidneys are one of the organs that must eliminate the mercury that poisons the kidney cells while they are filtering it out of the blood. Kidney disease is a huge industry in America. Treatment, drugs, dialysis, and transplants cost tens of BILLIONS of dollars every year. Could there be an economic reason not to eliminate mercury? Diseased kidneys that are removed should be analyzed for mercury content to see if it is a major contributor to the disease. Scientific studies have shown that kidneys are heavily contaminated with mercury as the body tries to cleanse itself.

Do you know that mercury can damage the heart? It can and does. Half of all deaths in this country are due to heart disease. Dentistry has helped this to be our number-one killer, yet few dentists believe that dentistry affects anything outside of the mouth. (The book *The Missing Link?* by Michael Ziff, D.D.S., discusses the mercury-heart connection.)

Do you know of anyone whose memory is slipping or who is experiencing a loss of feeling in their hands and feet? While not every health problem is caused by mercury poisoning, a large percent of them can be traced to mercury. A huge part of our health care costs may be from damage by dental materials placed by your well-meaning dentist. It is a scandal that is still going on.

Mercury Accumulates

Mercury is a cumulative poison; the longer it is in you, the more damaging it is. If you are ill with any of the problems listed as being caused by mercury, immediately find a dentist experienced in using composites and discuss having your fillings replaced.

The following case history is an example of the typical patient's attitude when they are placed between the ADA's misinformation and the medical attempts to resolve health problems that are likely related to mercury.

A middle-aged male patient with six old mercury fillings, including two which touch a gold crown, is typical of many patients. He has dental insurance and a good income. Having no fear of dental treatment, he has had several large mercury fillings replaced with composites in the past several years. He knows a little about the effects of mercury but does not seem to want to know more. He says he will replace the fillings if they have obvious decay or if something breaks.

That might be a reasonable position if there were no other problems, but the patient has arthritis in his shoulder joints and suffers from bone spurs that make movement painful. He has been told that mercury from fillings could be causing the chronic joint inflammation, which is a symptom of an autoimmune response commonly resulting from mercury toxicity. This inflammation can result in the formation of bone spurs. But he has taken no action to have the fillings replaced, but instead, has had surgery on one shoulder to physically remove the bone spurs. After three months he still had more pain from the surgery than he did from the bone spurs.

A more prudent course of action would be to remove the remaining mercury fillings and then try to reduce the mercury levels in the body on the strong chance that the inflammation will be reduced. It would seem that a bad experience with costly surgery would make an alternative treatment seem more attractive. Compare the cost of the shoulder surgery—$10 to $20,000 to try to remove a symptom (bone spurs) caused by a symptom (chronic inflammation), caused by mercury toxicity—with the cost of replacing the remaining metal dental work: the dental work would cost less than $2,000, and insurance would pay part of that.

If a dentist were to tell this patient that there was a fifty/fifty chance that cleaning out the metals from his mouth and tissues would end his bone spurs, the dentist could be charged with practicing medicine without a (medical) license. Even if the patient experienced a large improvement or a complete healing after having the metals removed, the dentist would still be considered guilty and risk losing his dental license. When dentists do get positive results from removing mercury fillings, the medical doctors and often the patients themselves attribute the improvement to other factors, such as "spontaneous remission."

This prevailing attitude keeps dentists from offering any help. Why would a dentist risk his ability to earn an income to help someone who does not want help? The attitude of most sick patients is that if dental materials really were the cause of so many problems, the government would have banned them long ago. Sure they would, just as they have done with cigarettes.

The FDA Avoids Going to The Public

Another example of the government turning its head from obviously hazardous procedures was exposed on a segment of "20/20," a TV news magazine. The show had a story about spinal operations in which screws were improperly used in tens of thousands of patients with heartbreaking results to many patients. This report said that these screws had not been approved by the FDA for use in spines. The FDA had even stated on two occasions that such use was wrong. Even so, the FDA had not banned this improper use. This irony prompted host Barbara Walters to ask, "Isn't the government supposed to protect us?"

Why do we think the government is protecting us from such hazards when its record is so bad? It has experimented on soldiers and citizens with radioactivity, syphilis, and plutonium. It routinely uses the first year of a new drug's release to the market to collect data on patient reactions, because it is too expensive to run large trials. Unfortunately, doctors do not always tell patients that all new drugs are still considered experimental. Many drugs are pulled off the market after the first year because of drastic, unexpected reactions. In the early 1990's the pharmaceutical giant Eli Lilly's new arthritis drug, Oraflex, proved to be fatal to many patients and was removed from use.

Other substances were on the market even longer before being banned. The sweetener cyclamate was banned as a cancer risk. Alar was banned for use on apples. But there are hundreds of additives and drugs that have been in use for years but have never been tested as they would be if they were new on the market. These products are designated by the FDA as category 1— "generally regarded as safe" or GRAS. When proof that they are not "safe" becomes overwhelming, these products are removed from the list and can no longer be used (in America). Unfortunately, during the years it takes the government to act on our behalf, thousands more people are damaged. This is not protection of the population, but protection of corporate America; Barbara Walters should know this.

FDA on Mercury Fillings

Mercury in fillings have never been approved by the FDA, which has avoided classifying amalgam at all. The FDA says mercury fillings are a "reaction product" made by dentists, and therefore it is the dentist's responsibility to assure the product's safety. Does that make you feel safe?

Stopping the placement of more mercury fillings is the first step in reducing the exposure of Americans to this hazard. The second step would be safely removing the mercury fillings from people's teeth; it will take a decade to accomplish this. There should be no room in the next century for mercury fillings and the damage they cause. If dentists will not listen to the truth, maybe it is time for the attorneys to get their attention. A half-dozen lawsuits per dentist would do it. Any dentist with half a brain should stop immediately and hope the statute of limitation runs out before lawyers catch on.

A Warning to Pro-Mercury Dentists

Listen, dentists, you are being warned. Stop this insanity or face the loss of all you own. Lawyers do not care if you are a nice guy who only meant to help people. They will say, "You, as a dentist, knew, or should have known, the effects of the materials you placed in your patient's body." There is no defense, because the FDA says you are the person who is ultimately responsible for the materials you use.

The legal reality is that the dentist stands alone. Soon, every patient with a mercury poisoning symptom may have an attorney. Win or lose, dentists could be spending their lives in court, not the office. Dentists could even win every suit and still have their lives ruined. And if one patient wins a single lawsuit, every mercury-using dentist's life would be a long series of court appearances. Malpractice insurance companies would go bankrupt, but the suits would go on. Dentists could lose everything they have.

There is a possible answer. Murray. J. Vimy, a well-respected Canadian dentist who researches the biological effects of mercury, suggests that an amnesty be declared for all dentists so they cannot be sued by patients for placing mercury fillings. He feels that the public will desperately ask these dentists to replace all the mercury fillings. (The same fillings they placed in the first place!) Amnesty may be possible, but dentists should not count on it. They should quit using mercury before it is too late.

The ADA'S Responsibility

The ADA is also responsible in its own way. As a trade organization composed mostly of dentists who use mercury, the ADA has no legal standing to promote or defend mercury use except as a trade group. It is a circular argument. Mercury-using dentists form a group which then says, "Mercury cannot harm you." When tobacco companies form groups that promote tobacco use, do you believe their statements about the safety of smoking? How many reports would it take to convince you that smoking is healthy?

The FDA Avoids Responsibility

Dentists cannot rely on the FDA to defend the use of mercury fillings because it has not approved their use. The most the agency has said is that it has not disapproved of their use, simply calling (once again) for "more studies" and leaving it at that. Until it decides to ban mercury, it becomes solely the dentist's responsibility when he mixes the powdered metals and mercury together and puts them in a patient's tooth. However, the FDA is not likely to ban mercury fillings any time soon because it has a history of being influenced by product manufacturers. Officials from the FDA commonly are hired as executives in pharmaceutical companies, and the expert witnesses they use are mostly connected to or work for these same companies. The movement of administrators at government agencies to the companies they regulate is so common it is called a "revolving door."

The bureaucrats who are the backbone of these agencies know that to stick their necks out would be career suicide. They know that they must "go along to get along."

To expect this cozy relationship between the FDA and the industries it regulates to change voluntarily is a pipe dream. It has been suggested that the long delay and huge amounts of money required to bring a new drug or medical device on the market is not to protect the public, but to give the companies already holding patents on similar products time to recoup their costs and make a profit before allowing the new competing products into the marketplace. This may sound cynical, but this possibility may be closer to the truth than we care to admit.

With regard to mercury fillings, both the ADA and the FDA have left themselves a way out. Instead of using the correct terms, "toxic" and "poisonous," they have said that there are a "few" people who are "allergic" to mercury. Using the milder term, "allergy," makes it sound like something one might have when they react to pollen or cat dander, instead of it being taken as the serious threat it is. The figure they use for the number of people affected has varied. They used two percent for a while, but found out that any health problem that affects two percent of the population is considered an epidemic. Currently, they have settled on one percent, which is still 2.5 MILLION people! A published study in 1969 in the *International Dental Journal* put the number at 22.5 percent, which would be 56 MILLION people!

Mercury Hypersensitivity

Even if only one percent of patients were hypersensitive, dentists should be obligated to check to see if their patients may be in that one percent. They should quit assuming that none of their patients are reactive to mercury because they do not see major outward signs, like breaking out in hives the next day. Do any dentists who use mercury run any type of tests before placing a filling? Not one! The only dentists who use compatibility tests are anti-mercury dentists. A dentist cannot say, "You already have mercury fillings, and you're still alive, so you must be all right," because the possibility of reaction to a substance increases the longer you are exposed and most of the reactions do not have obvious clinical signs, like hives. Mercury-using dentists probably do not even ask if their patients think they are allergic. They do not want to bring up the subject. If a patient asks them about mercury, they tend to become defensive, even angry.

The ADA may hope that it can suppress reaction to the information about the dangers of mercury until a material is invented that will be easy enough for any dentist to use. Remember, one of the reasons mercury fillings are used is that they are easy to put in. Not all dentists could change to a composite filling material that is more difficult to use; some speakers have conjectured that up to 40 percent of dentists do not have the physical skills necessary to place composites. That estimate seems to be too high, although a dentist anonymously wrote a book, *Dentistry and Its Victims*, in 1970, claiming that 30 percent of dentists were so incompetent that he called their type, "Dr. Poorwork."

Attacking Anti-Mercury Dentists

Maybe the ADA thinks calling anti-mercury dentists "quacks" will keep the truth buried. Calling anti-mercury dentists quacks is part of the "Big Lie" technique: If a lie is told often enough and loudly enough, people will believe it. The ADA has been using the technique to attack those dentists who disagree with its pro-mercury position rather than have a full forum of debate.

Since the ADA was formed by dentists who used mercury and is still composed mostly of pro-mercury dentists, is it any wonder that the association cannot admit that mercury is toxic and should not be used in people? If the ADA did confess that mercury was bad and apologized, as the national dental society has done in Sweden, such a confession would be equal to that of the communist leaders of the USSR, who after 70 years of rule, finally acknowledged that communism was not working and simply said something like, "We're sorry. We were wrong." Tens of millions were killed in the name of communism. Untold misery was caused. The people of the USSR knew that communism did not work because they had to live under its laws. But the powers that controlled them would not admit it. People who spoke out against the tyranny of the lies were called "dissidents" and were severely punished to keep them quiet.

Actually, the comparison is quite accurate. Tens of millions of people, maybe hundreds of millions, have been damaged by dental materials, their lives shortened or reduced in quality. Dentists who dare challenge the lies of the ADA are threatened with loss of their licenses to practice dentistry, an effective punishment that keeps most dentists quiet. Rules written into "codes of ethics" deny the right of free speech to dentists who dare tell their patients of the dangers of dental materials.

The denial of the right to free speech, even though guaranteed by the Constitution of the United States in the Bill of Rights, does not matter to the ADA as long as it can quiet dissent. But it will learn, as did the rulers of the USSR, that you cannot keep the truth suppressed forever. The lone dissenters are joining together. The people damaged by dentists are getting organized. The grass-roots support will keep growing until the truth is known by everyone.

Public Health Service Report on Mercury Fillings

In 1993 The Department of Health and Human Services' released a report called *Dental Amalgam*. It states: "The present effort is the first formal attempt by PHS (Public Health Service) to specifically focus on the benefits of dental amalgam use." "Benefits"? Does that sound as if their minds were made up in advance?

To show how pro-mercury these government agency personnel are, the Director of the National Institute of Dental Research, Dr. Harlod Loe (now retired), was chairperson of the Ad Hoc Subcommittee on the benefits of Dental Amalgam. In other words, the one person who should be leading the research toward safer dental materials is the leader of the group who backs the use of mercury. (This is the same dentist quoted earlier making statements that sounded like he was opposed to mercury fillings!) Do you think anyone against mercury would get a fair hearing with these agencies? Were the government leaders' minds made up from the beginning? Sure sounds that way!

One statement in this report denounces dentists who, "… are making bogus claims that dental amalgam (a mercury filling) is toxic or a causative agent for disease and, at the same time, promoting the replacement with other materials." In other words, if a dentist tries to help a patient get rid of mercury fillings that may be causing depression, the dentist can be attacked; this is just another attempt to keep anti-mercury dentists quiet, but it will not work because it is too late to hide the truth.

The report states elsewhere that "the toxicity of mercury and its compounds (that includes mercury fillings) have been recognized since antiquity and widely acknowledged in industry."

Does that sound like a safe material to you? The toxic effects of mercury have been known for thousands of years but the Department of Health and Services states that this report is about its "benefits."

Cost Involved In Replacing Mercury Fillings

The major benefit listed in the 1993 report for using dental amalgam was that it is easy for the dentist to use. But more important is the report's emphasis on the bottom line. Estimating that there are one billion mercury fillings in the mouths of Americans, one of the report's main points is that it would be too costly to replace them. This statement is an attempt to change the focus from a health issue to a money issue, but it is the health issue that is of primary importance. This is like saying that if a medical procedure causes mass poisoning, it is okay if it is cheap to do. Is that the kind of thinking you want from your National Institutes of Health?

The report goes on to estimate that about $250 billion would be needed to replace all of the billion mercury fillings. This sounds like a lot of money, but it must be viewed for what it is. If the number were true, it is just half the cost the "savings and loan bail out" and a quarter of the annual budget for "health" care. It is about the same amount of money it costs annually to pay for the overhead of the medical and dental insurance companies. Besides, this is a total cost for all the fillings, which could not be redone in one year, anyway. It may even take ten years at the rate of 100 million fillings per year, the amount of fillings currently done each year. Most importantly, of these 100 million fillings, 70 percent or more are replacement fillings. In other words, if dentists quit putting in new mercury fillings, the problem would solve itself in 10 years. Therefore, the cost of replacing all the fillings would not be an additional $250 billion, because the fillings will need to be replaced. The extra costs, the difference between using the poisonous mercury fillings or a safer filling material, the report estimated at only $10 billion a year, which is one-tenth of one percent of the total outlay of one TRILLION dollars spent for medical services. The cost comes to an average of $60 for every person who has mercury fillings. Therefore, the report's estimate on the cost of replacing the mercury fillings is misleading, inaccurate, and fictitious.

During all the cost analysis concerning replacing mercury fillings, nothing was figured for the savings when you do not have to treat people for the problems mercury causes. How much is spent treating mercury-caused depression? Arthritis? Alzheimer's disease? Heart disease? The savings from preventing the many common dental material-caused illnesses would more than pay for getting rid of the mercury fillings. If only 10 percent of all health problems are related to dental materials and techniques, correcting the problem could save a $100 billion every year from now on.

Another Call For More Research

The report does not deny that mercury fillings cause all the above noted problems, but simply states that same old refrain: "More research is needed." This is the common way for groups in power to buy time, while acting as if they really are concerned. More research may mean it would take another 10 or 20 years. It is not more information they want but more time. That may seem a reasonable risk unless it is YOUR health that has been ruined, unless it is YOUR parent that cannot remember their name, unless it YOUR wife's hands that are crippled with arthritis.

Considering the way this report has distorted the truth about the safety of mercury fillings, it shows that we cannot rely on the government to protect us. It is time to become more individually informed. It is time to end the old concept of dentistry based on the cheapest and easiest to use materials and begin to build a better future for dentistry based on our knowledge of what is true health.

History of Mercury Use in Dentistry

Mercury has been opposed as a toxic poison by some dentists ever since its introduction to America. In fact, there have been three "amalgam wars" in which anti-mercury dentists vigorously opposed its use. The first battle of the first "war" began when mercury first came to the U.S. from England in the 1830's. The opposition to mercury eventually waned, but it never was fully accepted by all dentists. Despite the early efforts to stop its use, mercury has prevailed because it has always been "economically useful" (meaning "cheap") for dentists to use. But it never was safe.

One of the pro-mercury arguments is that mercury has been used for 150 years. One would have hoped for some improvements in dentistry since before the Civil War. What would America look like if the architects bragged that they still use 150-year-old technology? The truth is that comparatively few mercury fillings were done before WWII. If you ask an older dentist what he did in the 1920's and 1930's, he would say mostly extractions. Most people ended their lives toothless. Unfortunately, there are no dentists from before the Civil War to tell us what dentistry was like before cheap sugar and expensive dental schools.

"The Second Amalgam War"

The "second amalgam war" was fought in the 1930's prior to WWII. The scientific studies were done in Germany. With the presence of anti-German feelings, it was easy to dismiss the research. In addition to the growing anti-Germany sentiment, another reason why the opposition to mercury went unheard was due to poor health. The average health of young Americans was not good in 1940, perhaps due to the Depression. Their teeth, in particular, were in poor condition due to poor diet. When the draft began for WWII, many were rejected because of poor teeth. Those that were accepted needed a lot of fillings. For lack of any other acceptable material, military dentists placed millions of mercury fillings which were fast and cheap. This huge increase in the number of mercury-filled teeth during the four years of the war may have been equal to all the teeth that had ever been filled with mercury in all years prior to WWII. Now the federal government has a vested interest in finding that mercury is safe. If mercury were banned because it causes problems, what would their responsibility be to the millions of servicemen in which it had placed mercury fillings? Do not forget that the military dentists are still placing mercury fillings and if the government said they were bad, they would have to change every one.

After WWII the rebuilding of Europe and the new booming economy made any worries about dental materials seem irrelevant. The military dentists returned to civilian life with much experience in using mercury fillings. There was the new anesthetic, novocaine, to control pain. The Depression was over. People had more money to spend on health care. Now dentists were able to fill almost any tooth using the mercury filling material.

Other Developments

More new equipment was developed. The hard carbide steel drill bits (burs) were invented, which did away with the old steel burs that required slow "grinding" in preparing a cavity because of their dullness. Ask people over 50 what it was like to get a filling done in the early 1950's.

The final breakthrough came with the ultrahigh speed drill. This new drill, using carbide steel burs, made it easy to create fillings. This combination of better anesthetics and the new drill with people's increasing incomes brought about the "golden age of dentistry," which ran from the late 1940's to the late 1960's. The reason the age was "golden" was that the demand for dental services exceeded the supply of dentists, so dentists were able to succeed financially without much effort or thought, particularly thoughts about the safety of mercury fillings.

So, the truth is that the vast majority of mercury fillings have been placed during a relatively short time period, from WWII to the present, only 50 years of common use, not the 150 years the ADA keeps mentioning. This time frame is critically important because mercury is built up slowly in the body. With our increased life spans there is now more time for the toxic effects of mercury to build up in our bodies. It is not at all surprising to see huge increases in the symptoms that have long been associated with chronic mercury poisoning. The disastrous effects of the "golden age of dentistry" are only now showing up in people. It was not a "golden age" at all, but a "mercury age."

"The Third Amalgam War"

The "third amalgam war" started in the 1970's and is still going on today. With more and more people, mostly outside of dentistry, recognizing the dangers of mercury fillings, this will be the last "war." The anti-mercury groups are prepared to fight until the end. After the ADA was forced to admit in 1980 that mercury did escape from fillings, many dentists expected that it would recommend that no more mercury fillings should be placed. But the ADA did not abandon mercury fillings, but actually became more in favor of their use. The organization also developed a rationale for not changing mercury fillings just to get the mercury out of your teeth by saying that removing fillings might damage the teeth conveniently forgetting that 70 percent or more of all fillings done are replacement fillings. In the years since the ADA admitted mercury escaped from fillings, there has been enough time that most all the mercury fillings could have been replaced if dentists had used non-mercury materials when they did routine replacement fillings and had quit placing new mercury fillings. Instead, because of their continued support of mercury, hundreds of millions, actually over a billion more of mercury fillings have been placed in people, many of whom have had the quality of their lives diminished by the toxic effects of mercury on their bodies.

The problems with mercury were scientifically proven to occur in the 1930's and yet, 70 years later, the facts are still being denied or discounted. This fraud of claiming mercury as safe has to stop; 70 years of suppression is enough. Patients deserve to have dentists use the best and safest dental materials. It is time to put aside the pre-Civil War materials and come out of the dark ages. It was bad then, and its continued use is wrong. The golden opportunity for the ADA to correct its mistake has passed. It is now time for the people to stop allowing dentists to use mercury in their mouths and to demand they use nontoxic materials.

Expansion of Mercury Fillings

The key physical characteristic of mercury that allows it to be used as a filling material is that it expands as it ages. This expansion is caused by corrosion which continues slowly over its life. Thus, the fillings locks itself into the cavity and helps seal the edges. Early mercury filling materials often expanded so much they split a tooth with painful results. The amount of expansion in current materials has been greatly reduced but mercury fillings still routinely put hairline cracks in the enamel. This is part of the reason cusps break off filled teeth. When mercury fillings are removed, internal cracks are routinely seen. Most dentist that notice them consider it a minor type of damage and may even think that the cracks are due to the natural breakdown of the teeth, conveniently giving them an effective, although untrue reason to sell the patient a crown.

Burnishing Fillings

In a mercury filling a type of polishing done by mechanically rubbing the surface of the mercury filling with pressure is done after the filling has set for at least one day. This technique smoothes the filling, making it shiny and can also be used on old fillings to make them look better and smooth off chipped edges caused by continuing expansion. What is really happening, however, is that fresh mercury is being pulled to the surface. This pull increases the free mercury near the surface, which is the mercury that comes out of the fillings and enters the body. This simple, but potentially harmful, procedure can be done by dental assistants and is sometimes referred to as an additional "profit center" for the dental practice. Thank goodness not many dentists do it because it is an extremely bad idea.

Another way fillings are burnished is by chewing. Mercury fillings in teeth subjected to chewing will have a shiny surface. This shine can be readily seen when non-chewing surfaces are viewed, which are normally black from oxidation (tarnishing).

EPA and OSHA On Mercury

The use of mercury in the dental office is controlled by rules and regulations under the state and federal offices of the Enviornmental Protection Agency (EPA) and the Occupational Safety and Health Administration (OSHA). Their rules cover such items as the allowable exposure levels of mercury vapor in the air, the method of cleanup for spilled mercury, and the disposal of any leftover mercury filling material called "mercury scrap." This mercury scrap can be from new filling or pieces of old fillings that are not sucked into the sewer line. This scrap must be handled in specified ways to keep mercury from escaping into the air as vapor. It seems that the EPA believes the only safe place to store mercury filling material is in people's teeth.

Delany Clause

For any product that caused even the smallest increase in cancer risk, the FDA is required by law to implement the Delaney Clause which requires an immediate ban. This clause was used to get rid of cyclamates and many food colors in the 1970's and 1980's. But now the clause is being ignored, while the FDA tries to have Congress change its power by allowing products that show some only small increases in the cancer rate to be sold and used. This move is based on the concept that there is a monetary limit when it comes to saving lives that a product with some benefits should stay on the market, as long as it does not kill too many people. That mindset should tell you who rates higher with the FDA, you or industry.

Remember, if you have a tooth removed that has a mercury filling in it, according to EPA and OSHA regulations, the dentist cannot give it to you, but must dispose of it in an appropriate way. One minute it is safe in your mouth and the next minute it is a threat to all humanity. This inconsistency in regulations shows that you cannot rely on the federal government to protect your interests. You must protect yourself.

Difficulty in Disposal

After extraction of a tooth, a dentist cannot throw the tooth in the trash until it is sterilized, but if it contains a mercury filling, it cannot be sterilized because the high heat and pressure will cause a release of mercury vapor. The mercury filling could be cut out with a drill, but that gives off extra vapor, plus puts more mercury in the sewer and, in reality, there still will be some mercury left in the tooth structure to vaporize. There is no answer that does not make things worse.

The problem with what the dentist should do with the scrap mercury is perplexing. It is recommended that the dentist store the scrap mercury in closed container filled with an X-ray developing chemical, then occasionally sell it to a mercury recycling firm. Unfortunately, in the 1980's a few dentists who sold their scrap to a legitimate recycling firm found themselves subject to $70,000 fines. It seems that the firm had gone bankrupt before the EPA found that they had contaminated the soil around their processing plant. Since the EPA could no longer fine the firm, they sued the dentists. The mercury scrap is not valuable enough for any dentist to take such a risk.

So where does the mercury scrap go? If the mercury coming out of dental offices were traced, it would be found that it is going everywhere, and with mercury, because of its toxicity, there are no safe places. The scrap mercury goes to landfills, to hazardous trash pickup services (which may burn it), down sewer lines, to recyclers, or it may be accumulated until retirement, then buried or just left in the corner of a basement. Perhaps, since the ADA thinks this material is so safe, it should be sent to ADA headquarters. Unfortunately, it is too toxic to send through the mail!

With all these precautions you would think dentists would be reluctant to put mercury into someone's mouth. It is beyond reason that dentists do not see the inconsistency in using mercury in their patients while protecting themselves from exposure. Luckily, the number of mercury fillings is declining; there were ONLY 100 MILLION done last year.

Pregnancy and Dentistry

There is growing concern about the effects of dental materials and procedures on the developing fetus. Birth defects from mercury are well-known and cannot be challenged even by the most ignorant pro-mercury advocate. The first damaging effect dental materials may have occurs even before pregnancy to the sperm or egg, damaging the genetic code or even making fertilization impossible. This may be one of the reasons for the 50 percent decrease in male fertility that has happened in last 50 years. Most of the real damage happens when the fertilized egg is exposed to mercury, although mercury can easily cross the placental barrier and be absorbed by the developing fetus. In fact, the concentration of mercury may be higher in the embryo than in the mother.

In response to this hazard many European countries have stopped the use of mercury fillings in pregnant women and children under six. In 1994 a California court ruled that a dentist who places mercury fillings must post a sign warning patients of birth defects which may be caused by mercury to state: "This office uses amalgam filling material which contain and expose you to mercury, a chemical known to the State of California to cause birth defects and other reproductive harm. Please consult your dentist for more information."

A federal court at first overturned the lower court, but it in turn was overturned, so the ruling stands. Has it been effective? Probably not, as nothing seems to have happened. Other court orders to the California Dental Board concerning telling the people of California the truth about mercury have not been followed as the mercury-using dentists resist self-incrimination.

Such efforts only delay the inevitable, but it is patients who pay with their declining health.

The First Six Weeks

The most critical time in the formation of a fetus is the first six weeks, when all of the basic organ systems are developing. Damage that occurs then can be life-threatening and disfiguring, examples being cleft palates and spina bifida (malformation of the spinal column). The absorbed mercury is attracted to the embryo's developing central nervous system, which has been shown to lead to a higher incidence of cerebral palsy.

Dentists should routinely ask their female patients of childbearing age if they are pregnant each time they are seen. If a woman wants to have her mercury fillings replaced, it is best to delay conception for six months after the replacement of her mercury fillings to give her body time to begin to detox. This process should minimize the risk to an upcoming pregnancy because mercury levels can temporarily rise after filling replacement. A woman should NEVER have mercury fillings removed or placed while pregnant or nursing. In nursing mothers, mercury is passed to the baby through the mother's milk, even showing higher concentrations in the infant than in the mother.

In fact, it is recommended that a woman have no dental work at all while she is pregnant. A rare exception may be made to allow teeth cleaning, but only for only someone with a serious gum problem, one involving infection and pain. Routine cleanings should not be done because even they can produce a "septicemia" (bacteria in the blood). Any time there is bleeding, even from brushing, mouth bacteria are able to enter the body and be carried throughout the body by the blood stream. Any blood-borne bacteria are potential risks to the embryo or fetus. Such a risk is not warranted for any routine dental procedure.

Emergency problems during pregnancy must be judged individually. Most filling emergencies can be handled by the use of temporary filling materials. Extractions of infected teeth need to be coordinated with the woman's physician. Antibiotics should be used cautiously because the fetus may be negatively affected by antigens from the mother or by developing antibiotic-resistant bacteria. In an ideal world a woman should be healthy before getting pregnant and that includes a healthy mouth.

Damage to Dentists' Children

An example of how easy it is to dismiss the dangers of mercury in children is that of a pro-mercury dentist who wrote a "letter to the editor" of JADA claiming he had personal proof that mercury use was all right. He said his oldest child, a teenage boy, had several mercury fillings and no health problems, but his young daughter did not have any mercury fillings but had serious health problems; unfortunately, he may be wrong about both of them. Although the older boy may appear healthy now, he is building up mercury in his tissues because mercury accumulates over the length of the exposure; therefore, he may not exhibit any health problems until much later.

On the other hand, his daughter may have been damaged genetically by exposure to mercury even before conception through the dentist's exposure to mercury in his office. Or she could have been damaged during development by mercury contamination from her mother's fillings (if she had any). Or he may have inadvertently brought mercury home from his office on his clothes. OSHA now requires that dental staff change clothes and clean them at the office to prevent contamination in their personal washing machines.

It is also well-documented that the children of dentists and their staffs have a higher incidence of genetic damage. A higher rate of spontaneous abortions is also reported. If, in fact, his daughter's health problems were caused by her early exposure to mercury, it would be a sorry legacy to give her. But his denial may bring about the same legacy for many of his patients. Dentists have much to answer for because their "defiant ignorance" on the issue of mercury in fillings has brought lifelong despair to so many.

Birth Defects Warning

Besides mercury, other metals can cause damage to developing embryos. Nickel, a dangerous metal, is used routinely in our children, mainly for braces and crowns. It would be an unreasonable risk to have braces just before or during pregnancy. Remember, genetic damage is permanent. It is strongly recommended that a woman be mercury-free and nickel-free at least six months before attempting to get pregnant.

Safety Lights in Running Shoes

Another new concern about mercury has been raised with regard to the safety of lighted running shoes. The small lights that make runners safer by making them more visible at night may be unsafe for the environment, because many of these shoes use a "mercury" switch to turn the lights on and off. The mercury is sealed so it is not a threat to the wearer, but it may be a threat to the environment when the shoes are thrown away. The use of mercury in these shoes may violate some state laws, and these states are worried because millions of pairs of these shoes have been sold.

The manufacturers have said that the amount of mercury is small, "just a bead." The concern is how much mercury is in the "beads" in five million pairs that have been sold? According to a shoe company report there is one gram of mercury per pair, which came to 15,400 pounds or 7.7 tons. Maybe the authorities should be worried. Pollution experts were quoted in news releases to have warned: "It is estimated that the amount of mercury on a pinhead, once airborne, is enough to cause a fish advisory on a 40-acre lake. Mercury is a toxic chemical that has been the particular focus of cleanup efforts worldwide." Subsequently, the shoe manufacturer has come to an agreement with the State of Minnesota to pay monetary damages, do educational advertising, and to offer a postage-paid return envelope so anyone who bought the shoes can send them back when the shoes are worn out.

What about the mercury in the fillings in the mouths of the citizens of Minnesota? How much mercury is in an average filling? It is difficult to give an exact amount of mercury contained in one filling because the amount of mercury is not given by weight. The leading text on dental materials does not discuss the weight of the mercury, only the proportion, but it would be a large filling to contain a gram of mercury. It has been estimated that the total dental use of mercury per year is 60 tons, down from 100 tons a few years ago. It is impossible to estimate the total amount of mercury in the teeth of 150 million Americans or the total amount used over the last 50 years.

Mercury is 13.9 times as dense as water, which means that a two-liter bottle full of mercury would weigh 26 pounds. The amount of mercury in that bottle would be enough for 11,832 pairs of shoes and the amount of mercury in five million pairs of shoes would fill 592 two liter bottles. That is a lot of mercury!

Crematoriums

It has been reported in the newspaper that 25 percent of the mercury pollution in the air in Denmark is from crematoriums. Surely, it is also a problem here in the U.S., but one that people tend to avoid discussing. Most people do not want to know if the air they are breathing is filled with "stuff" from a crematorium.

There are only a few solutions to the problem. We could stop cremation, we could filter the exhaust from the crematoriums or we could require that the teeth be removed from the bodies before cremation. The later solution would be ironic, because the problem that caused the death in the first place might have been solved by removing the toxic metal while the person was still alive.

The issue of air pollution from mercury being burned during cremation brings up another environmental concern. Are there toxic metals left in the "ashes?" If they are, what precautions should be taken in their disposal? Are they safe without being sealed? Are they safe even if sealed?

Of course, cemeteries are filled with deceased people who have mercury fillings and who are lying in lead-lined caskets. Cemeteries may be the most toxic "landfills" around. Not an environmental problem now, but will it be in a century or two?

There is another place has high levels of mercury--vapor in the air in dental offices. The standard dental school text, *Science of Dental Materials*, states that one dental office in ten exceeds the limit for mercury vapor. The book recommends yearly monitoring, which is rarely, if ever, done by any office. That may not be a major concern for patients who are not in the office long but could be for the dentists and their staffs.

Sewers

All dental offices have central vacuum systems, which create the suction for the wands that suck the water, saliva, and debris from dental treatments out of your mouth: A small one called a saliva ejector and a large one called a high-volume evacuator. Suction is created by a vacuum pump, which pulls the various materials from your mouth through a disposable tip into a system of pipes which lead to the pump, which then expels it all into the sewer line. In most offices this sewer line connects to the city sewer system. Dentists do not want to discuss what happens to the material the vacuum sucks out of your mouth because it is full of toxic metals and potentially hazardous biological wastes.

Sewers are not the nicest of places, anyway, but the people who work in them are at considerable risk. Not only are they exposed to every germ that infects humans, but also to the mercury flushed out of dental offices into these sewers. Primitive traps in the vacuum lines in dental offices catch some of the larger pieces, but this may be only a small percentage of all that passes through; the rest goes out to the sewer. This process will change as the EPA is more concerned with the mercury in the environment than the ADA is about the mercury in your mouth.

Many of the heavier metal pieces may settle into cracks and seams in the sewer pipes, which may make working on these pipes very dangerous. The rest ends up in a sewage treatment plant, ending up as a contaminant in the sludge or escapes with the treated water downstream to the next city. Either way, it is an environmental toxin which will contaminate the fish and other animals, plus the vegetation and soil. The mercury can never be broken down because it is an element, which means it is as small as it can get. Once mercury enters the environment, it is very hard, if not impossible, to get rid of it.

Official Reaction

The ADA is well-aware of this problem. In the early 1990's officials in Tucson, Arizona, closed many dental offices in an attempt to stop mercury from entering the sewers. They were defeated in court by the ADA because they did not have any "studies" showing what amount would be considered unsafe. (There is that technique again by which you can ignore a problem by calling for studies.) In a subsequent national meeting on the problem a consensus to research guidelines was reached that can be set up nationally; this will delay any action well into the future.

The Japanese government has banned mercury fillings in at least one dental school because of mercury getting into the sewer. Mercury is also an environmental concern in European countries. (They do have studies, but probably studies the ADA would conveniently find unacceptable.) Dental offices in some European countries are required to have mercury separators on their sewer lines. Although these devices are commercially made and are available in this country, dentists will not install them voluntarily and they will have to be made a requirement. If the ADA has its way, once guidelines are established, the adoption of the guidelines will be fought city by city.

One would think that the admission that there is a problem with mercury in the sewer discharge from dental offices would mean that there is a problem with the use of mercury in the mouth. It is still like "the emperor's new clothes" when everyone is looking at the truth but no one believes what they are seeing so they pretend that there is no problem.

Microwave Theory

Recently, an interesting theory about the increase in problems caused by mercury has been raised. Due to the tremendous increase in microwave transmissions in the last decade, each of us is constantly bombarded with microwaves. Generally they pass right through us, but do not pass through metal, including mercury fillings. The mercury, not being firmly bound to the filling, could be caused to come out of the fillings if hit by a microwave. This idea sounds far-fetched at first, but think about what happens if you place a metal object in a microwave oven. (Don't try it.) It creates sparks and can ruin the unit. Why wouldn't the same thing happen, with less intensity, to a metal filling?

Consider this example of the possible effects of microwave energy on mercury fillings: During a TV show about parachuting off a microwave transmission tower, one of the experienced jumpers warned the new person about spending more than six minutes on top of the tower. He said the microwaves were so powerful that your fillings would heat up! Now most of us are not going to be spending any time on top of a 1200-foot microwave tower, but this example suggests that microwaves do have an effect on dental metals, including mercury. Maybe this theory merits some research, as we are being exposed to more and more microwave radiation.

Risk From The Dental Use of Mercury

The concept that mercury fillings have been widely used for over a century may seem to make mercury an unlikely candidate for causing a "new" disease. But in reality, the majority of mercury fillings have been placed since 1940. That time period coincides perfectly with the appearance of Alzheimer's sufferers. A 50-year, low-level exposure to mercury fillings allows mercury to slowly build up in the brain. By then the brain cells become so damaged that symptoms appear. The longer people are exposed, the more severe the effect.

Many older people no longer have teeth, but even people without teeth may have been exposed to high levels of mercury earlier in their life, perhaps while playing with mercury as children. Dentists used to give small amounts of mercury to children to take home. It was fun to play with "quicksilver." Eventually, the mercury would be "lost," maybe in the rug or in cracks in the floor. This "lost" mercury would contaminant the air for years. Nowadays, under OSHA regulations, the amount of mercury in a thermometer, if spilled, would require the area to be vacated and special cleanup procedures initiated.

It is entirely within the realm of possibility that mercury is the cause of Alzheimer's. It will be a sorry legacy if all the good intentions of the dental profession end up destroying millions of lives. Maybe spending a bit more to have non-mercury fillings or even having your mercury fillings removed seems like a good idea. Does waiting 10 to 20 more years for the results of the current studies seem reasonable? If the past is any indication, if these studies show mercury is a causal agent in Alzheimer's, the "powers that be" will challenge their validity, claiming that the studies are "flawed" and will call for still more research. How long are you willing to wait? It is your choice.

Testing for Mercury

Many people are concerned about having mercury poisoning. They ask their physician to test them. Since the physicians are not knowledgeable about mercury build-up in the body they do the most obvious test which is a urine test. For mercury to show in the urine, it would have to be floating freely in the blood so it could be filtered by the kidneys. Mercury is so active it does not stay in the blood but attaches itself to the cell walls or enters the cells. A low number is usually the result and the patient is told they do not have a mercury problem when they may be the most at risk people.

The correct way is to do the test twice. The second time the patient is given a mercury chelator (bonding) drug, (dimercapto-propane sulfonic (DMPS) acid), which pulls the mercury out of its hiding places. If the patient has a lot of mercury the second test will show a much higher reading. Only physicians familiar with mercury problems will know to use this technique.

The Role of Mercury Filling in Resistance to Antibiotics

A study published in 1993 states that mercury fillings can cause bacteria in the intestine to become resistant to antibiotics. The exposure to mercury leaking out of the fillings created mutated bacteria that were able to resist being hurt by further exposure to mercury. Although that may sound good for the bacteria, the bad news is that the same genes that protected the bacteria from the toxic mercury made them resistant to antibiotics. Obviously, this may pose a major problem for the 150 million Americans who have mercury fillings and could be critical for many people whose lives depend on stopping a life-threatening infection.

Resistance of bacteria to antibiotics would put us back into the dangerous pre-penicillin world. Before penicillin became available during WWII, a minor scratch, let alone a major wound, could lead to death by gross infection. Now, the newspapers frequently report on the new strains of antibiotic-resistant bacteria, such as some strains of staphylococcus, tuberculosis, and some venereal diseases that are spreading through certain segments of the population. These reports include the dreaded Strep A, which has been labeled the "flesh-eating" germ that causes rapid and hard-to-stop infections.

Another Mode of Developing Resistance

Another source of resistant bacteria is in the new concept of treating gum disease. Small dressings containing low levels of antibiotics are placed around teeth with gum infections. Initially, this treatment will reduce the population of bacteria, but after repeated use, the bacteria will become resistant. Ironically, the initial gum inflammation may be caused by a toxic reaction to the patient's mercury fillings.

One of the most important measures you can take to help prevent antibiotic-resistant bacteria from developing in you or your family is not to have any mercury fillings placed. Another way you can protect yourself and your family is to avoid the casual use of antibiotics. If you use antibiotics once a year, it is too often. You are risking developing resistant bacteria, as well as an allergic reaction. It is possible that using antibiotics for minor infections may mean that you will not be able to use them in a true emergency. While it is true that new antibiotics are being developed, they are also becoming more toxic to the patient, not just the bacteria, and are very expensive.

Natural Resistance of The Immune System

Antibiotics may weaken our immune systems in another way that is rarely discussed. Our immune systems develop as we grow because they get stronger with use. When Europeans first came to the Americas, they devastated the native populations with diseases to which the Europeans had developed resistance. A million or more native people died from these infections. But have you heard of Europeans dying from infections from the native people?

Why were the native people so vulnerable? It was because they were not exposed to these germs and they did not live in the squalid cities so common in Europe. These awful conditions created Europeans who were naturally resistant. Those that did not develop resistance died and did not pass on their genes.

We use antibiotics to quicken the defeat of invading bacteria. By this use we take away the natural way our immune systems develop strength. It may seem like a hard way to look at things saying we must suffer some for our immune systems to develop, but that is the truth. Antibiotics should only be used when there are no other options, not as the first option.

Vaccinations also weaken our immune systems in a similar manner. While there can be a case made for the use of vaccines for life-threatening illnesses, the trend is to use them for every germ. The new one for chicken pox will be a good example of a disease that should be let run its course. We will reap a legacy of adult chicken pox and other similar infections, such as shingles, from the use of this vaccine.

Many vaccines contain Thimersol as a preservative. Thimersol is a mercury compound we are injecting into our babies. Our ignorance knows no bounds!

We are seeing in our country a rapid increase in autoimmune problems that may be traced to our misuse of medicines, such as antibiotics. We must be more respectful of our immune systems, learn to strengthen them, not weaken them. Our insistence in treating symptoms dooms us to a future where autoimmune problems lessen the quality of our lives.

Alzheimer's Disease

Twenty years ago no one had heard of Alzheimer's disease; now it is a leading cause of death in older Americans, and its incidence seems to be growing. This disease's effects on families is devastating both emotionally and financially

Intelligent, educated people are reduced to infancy. Costs for home care may reach $20,000 a year, which is not covered by government or private health insurance plans. This is a sad situation, but what does it have to do with dentistry? Aluminum has been mentioned as a possible cause of Alzheimer's because it is found in the brain tissue of deceased victims. Many "experts" disagree. Recently, mercury has been discovered in the brain tissue of Alzheimer's patients.

You would think that mercury would have been suspected as a cause from the beginning. It is well-known that mercury is attracted to nerve cells and the brain (central nervous system). In the disaster at Minamata Bay in Japan, mercury-contaminated wastewater was released into the water of Minamata Bay, contaminating fish and poisoning the people who ate them. Later, scores of babies were born physically deformed and severely brain damaged. A similar contamination of people occurred in Iraq, where seeds coated with mercury containing fungicides were mistakenly used for flour. Babies born to several of the pregnant women who ate the flour suffered severe brain damage.

Mercury and Alzheimer's Disease

Mercury loves nerve tissue, and the brain is all nerve tissue. It should come no surprise that mercury is always found in the brains of Alzheimer's Disease patients. Does it cause the disease? It is hard to prove since the government frowns on giving mercury to patients to see if they get Alzheimer's Disease. Without doing human experimentation, the best that can be done is to study how mercury affects animals and through autopsies of human brains.

Dr. Boyd Haley, a professor at the University of Kentucky in Lexington, has been testing the connection between Alzheimer's and mercury. The number of fillings corresponds to the amount of mercury found in the brain; the more fillings, the more mercury is found. Once the mercury is in the brain, it is hard to remove. Dr. Haley believes dental materials are poisoning millions of Americans. He also has been testing the toxicity of root-canals on enzyme systems. His findings in both areas are alarming.

These findings do not surprise researchers in toxicology because they have known the dangers of dental metals for decades. Thousands of research papers show the dangers but they are uniformly ignored by the ADA and dentists. The media do not seem interested as most of their stories are sent by the ADA and not from their own investigations. The media reports are mostly self-serving puff-pieces extolling the virtues of the establishment. The truth is available in libraries and throughout the Internet. You must look for the truth because it is not in ADA's and dentists' best economic interests to tell you, but is in your best interest.

The Caduceus and the God Mercury

The Roman god, Mercury, is depicted as having wings on his feet, wearing a helmet, and carrying a small staff intertwined with two snakes. The staff, called a "caduceus," which comes from the Greek word for messenger, was adopted as the symbol of medicine and dentistry. Although it is said to represent high ideals such as good health, caring, and hope, unfortunately, the values the god Mercury really represented were commerce, property, and wealth; maybe they do reflect the values of many in the "healing" professions, after all.

The god Mercury had other traits. He was considered "rather crafty and deceptive, and even as being a trickster or thief" not the kind of qualities wanted in any profession. The caduceus is one more way the profession of dentistry is tied to the metal mercury. Perhaps the profession would be better off if it dropped both the caduceus and the use of mercury to rid itself of all connections to this poisonous metal.

The Costs of Having Mercury Replaced

There are many costs involved in replacing mercury fillings and other toxic metals. The simplest cost is financial. If only fillings are involved and you have a composite filling done to replace each mercury filling, the total cost may range from $1000 to $3000 or more. That amount may be a lot compared to what people usually spend for dental care in a year, but compared to medical costs, it is quite reasonable. In today's medical system it is easy to run up $1000 in costs for a sprained ankle.

Dental work may also seem like a bargain when compared to the new multiple sclerosis drug that costs $10,000 per year, or the $15,000 in costs to remove a kidney stone, or the $50,000 needed for a heart bypass that may not help at all. But you may reply, "Insurance pays for those things!" Insurance does not pay for anything! YOU DO! You pay for the insurance, which is really prepaid medical bills or have you not noticed that $4000 per year being taken out of your paycheck?

Or compare the cost of dental work to other common purchases. When the average house costs $120,000 and the average car sells for $15,000 to $20,000, the cost of a mouthful of new dental work seems reasonable. As with the new home or car you may want to spread the costs of your dental work over several years by getting a loan.

You may feel that because the dentist has put this "junk" in your mouth, he should take it out at no charge. However, the majority of dentists would probably decline. Your only way of pursuing that is through legal means. Unfortunately, the only people who will be able to get us out of this toxic wasteland are the same dentists who got us into it.

It is frustrating to have to pay for something twice. Many patients have had recent dental work done that then needs to be replaced. It may happen that part of the first work was paid for by a dental plan, but since the plan will not cover the same work if it is redone within a year, the whole cost of the new work must be borne by the patient. While much of these costs may seem unfair, the patient must keep in mind whose problem it is and who must solve it. The dentist who placed the previous work may be to blame, at least morally, but if the patient spends his energy blaming others, he may have to pay a much higher price emotionally. It may be best to accept what has to be done, find a way to do it, and then spend the energy in correcting the problem.

Emotional Costs

This emotional component can also show up in other ways. This component may show up as a reluctance to have work done because of leftover fear from a bad childhood experience or simply the frustration of having to sit still while the work is being done in your mouth. Whatever the reason, the patient must deal with it, hopefully with some help from an empathetic dental staff. Treatment can be a more pleasant experience if the patient and staff work together to make it as tolerable an experience as possible.

Your cooperation is essential for a good outcome. It is not a matter of just letting the dentist do what must be done, even though you may not like it. Your positive attitude helps the treatment to be a combined effort, because when the patient is fully cooperative, the dentist can do his best work. If he must spend his energy overcoming your resistance, he cannot focus on the technical work to be done.

Much patient resistance is due to the fear of the unknown. If you make sure that you are fully informed, the treatment will make more sense; as it loses its mystery, you lose your fear. Learn about what is being done by asking questions of the dentist and staff.

Familiarity Breeds Acceptance

The following case history illustrates how initial resistance to treatment fades as comfort levels increase:

A young man who wanted his mercury fillings replaced because he thought it was best not to have mercury in his teeth was so apprehensive at first that he delayed beginning treatment for two years. He finally overcame his initial fear by thoroughly discussing the procedure with his dentist, but his apprehension was still so high only one quadrant was finished during his appointment instead of the planned two quadrants. Fortunately, he gained confidence during the first appointment that having the work done was not going to be as hard or uncomfortable as he had anticipated.

The second appointment went easily for him and two more quadrants were completed, leaving only the quadrant not done the during the first appointment to be finished. By the end of the third appointment the patient was so relaxed that he fell asleep during treatment! It is common for most patients to experience a similar pattern. The actual dental work is usually less traumatic than patients anticipate. In fact, it is the cooperation of the patient that can either make a procedure simple or difficult, and the less resistance the dentist has to cope with the better his work will be.

For some people, however, the emotional component is complicated by waiting so long to have the toxic material removed that they must also confront the expense of illnesses associated with these toxins. Many sick people have exhausted themselves financially, as well as physically and emotionally, trying to find a medical cure from "dental-caused" illnesses. Ill people have little emotional reserves and having a lot of dental work done in a short time can be an ordeal. Even if it takes only eight hours of treatment, they may anticipate it as if it were 800 hours. But as with most fears, the reality is not as bad as what was anticipated.

Unexpected Reaction

In another case a thirty-year-old, athletic woman wanted her mercury out. She had been fighting many health problems that no one had been able to solve. Because she had had limited dental work done in the last 15 years, she was nervous, even jumpy. After the first hour of her first appointment she had visibly

147

relaxed. The anxiety that she had built up melted in the face of the reality. The treatments were not painful or frightening, as she had feared.

After her second hour she was even more relaxed. Then she noticed that she was able to make a tight fist with her left hand, something she had been unable to do when she began the mercury removal two hours earlier. Such rapid improvements were probably due to the elimination of the galvanic currents (electricity) the metal fillings had been generating. These changes, which seem to affect parts of the body far from the mouth, tend to verify the far-reaching effects of dental materials.

Waiting Too Long

Other people may end up paying the ultimate price for waiting to have their toxic metal removed from their mouths. In another case an older man, an outdoor, robust type, visited the dentist because he was full of toxic metals. He was worried about losing what level of health he had. He had most of his teeth but over the years they had become full of mercury fillings; plus he had crowns, bridges, and root-canals. He had had so much dental work that there was no way to "fix" his teeth. So the dentist told him that the only way he could get rid of all that dental "stuff" was to have his teeth removed and dentures made. To go from a mouthful of "something" to a set of dentures is a drastic step, both dentally and emotionally. Understandably, he did not want to go to that extreme.

Many people facing the loss of parts of their body will choose to "go out" in one piece, particularly when you cannot be sure that such drastic treatment will be in time to help. The ordeal of enduring multiple extractions and learning to use dentures was beyond what he was willing to do.

He became hostile because he still felt robust and concluded for himself that such treatment was unnecessary. In fact, he said he was in such good shape that he would outlive the dentist. The dentist hoped he could continue to maintain his health in spite of the mess of toxic dental materials in his body. He did not. He only lived about 18 more months. And, unfortunately, he probably would not have changed his mind if he could have been guaranteed 10 extra years!

Becoming One With Your Disease

Other people get into a relationship with their diseases. Their disease take so much of their time and energy that they do not know how to live without. Over many years the disease even becomes the basis of their relationships with their spouse, family, doctors, and friends, many of whom may share the same disease.

A cure changes everything. Many people cannot handle that much change; therefore, they resist treatment. Although it sounds strange, it is a common problem, a psychological trap that can snare any of us. Because so many people accept declining health as their lot in life, one of the true costs of toxic dental work is ruined health. It does not have to be this way, and much of it is due to our attitude.

However, even the right attitude toward removing toxic material can slip away. A sporadic patient, one who would only come in when she had a problem, eventually had all her mercury fillings replaced over 10 years. One day she came into our office with a broken filling. When the dentist noticed a new mercury

149

filling, she said it had been done while he had been on vacation. When the dentist asked her why she had let the other dentist place a mercury filling after having all her other ones replaced, she said the other dentist told her it would be cheaper. Then she added a saying common in the area, "Poor people have poor ways."

That phrase shows an attitude that is hard to overcome. The saying is not true because many poor people do not have poor ways and many "well-off" people do. It would be better to say, "Ignorant people have ignorant ways." Fortunately, ignorance is a curable problem. One only has to learn, ask questions, and think. It requires no money. To blame a lack of money is to trap oneself mentally. Do not condemn yourself by thinking "poor," when the true cost of toxic dental work is paid for in ruined health.

As you can see, there are many costs to be considered. It is much easier for a well person to get their dental work done than to wait until they are sick and then try to get well. Often, by the time someone's health fails, it is too hard to regain it. Be smart and do not delay getting your mouth cleaned of all poisonous metals.

Falling Off The Mercury-Free Wagon

A patient from Idaho came to have his mouth checked for problems. He had had his mercury fillings out but a dentist had placed a new one. It seemed strange that a person who had his fillings removed for health reasons would then have another one placed. When asked, he said that he told the dentist he wanted a composite and the dentist said he would place one. Then after the cavity preparation was done, the dentist told him it was too large for a composite and he would have to place a mercury filling. The patient, being in a bad position, let the dentist do it. This treatment is a common problem.

The mercury filling was removed and the cavity was found to be rather small and did not have any problems that would have stopped even a poorly skilled dentist from putting in a composite. It must be considered that the dentist never planned to follow the patient's request. People must remember that dentistry is an elective service and they have every right to get what they want. The patient had the right to tell the dentist "No!" He might have said, "If you do not feel qualified to complete the work as we agreed, then you must place a temporary filling and I will not pay anything for your services."

You never have to let a dentist to impose on you anything you do not want. In a legal sense, he had a contract with the dentist to do a particular service. The dentist's failure to deliver as agreed is a violation of the contract and no payment is required. There might even be grounds for damages but the cost of collecting them would not be worth it. If the dentist would threaten to sue you or file insurance that is not correct you can file complaints with your insurance company or with your state attorney general. As a consumer, you must stand up for your rights in these situations and not cave into feelings of intimidation.

There are cases where the patient may be wrong, so use common sense. Realize that many people who are sick and have been through years of doctor treatments can be less-than-ideal patients. It is important to ask your questions before treatment begins, even before treatments are scheduled. Once you have decided to proceed, than try to be as cooperative as possible. The dentist does have the right to tell you that you are being too much of a pain or charge you extra to compensate for time it takes to handle delays.

Detoxification

An important factor in reducing the emotional costs of having mercury replacement fillings is staying focused on the goal of becoming healthier. When those black mercury fillings are viewed for what they are, toxic metals implanted in your body, looking forward to their removal becomes easy. After learning of the dangers of mercury fillings, many patients come to hate them and want them out instantly. It is common for patients to want to start immediately.

However, do not expect miracles; they have happened, but not to everyone. For every year the toxins have been implanted, it may take your body a month to detox itself. If the metals have been in 20 or 30 years, expect it to take 20 or 30 months to get the majority of the mercury out of the body's tissues. It may be impossible to get it completely out of every cell in the body.

Detoxification is the process of removing the poisonous materials people have absorbed from dental materials and other sources, such as, food, medicines, and the environment. Since dentists have helped put these toxins in people, it is reasonable that they should be able to help them get rid of them. It is not seen that way by the dental and medical boards. If a dentist tries to remove toxins, he could be accused of practicing medicine without a license. The best of both worlds would be if dentists could work with physicians who do detoxification.

The major type of detoxification is called intravenous chelation (chemical bonding to remove metals). One or more of a large variety of chelation agents are put into the patient via an IV over an hour or two, often done as support before, during, or after a dental appointment or after all the dental metals are out. While many agents can be used, the best are vitamin C and glutathione. What is used needs to be determined by the physician doing it and not by the dentist.

Most patients do not go as far as having chelation done, an additional expense at a time when patients are trying to handle the costs of the dental treatment. If using a chelating physician is not possible, it is still a good idea to do help the body get rid of its toxic load.

The sicker a person is, the slower you must go so you do not overwhelm your body. Getting better is the goal, not getting sicker. Depending on your state of health, you can choose from many methods of detoxification. Detoxification using vitamins, herbs, homeopathics (only with the help of a trained practitioner), amino acids, and therapies such as, a sauna bath, can speed your recovery.

The problem with detoxing is that you can do it too fast; when this happens your symptoms get worse as the metals are released into the blood. Not all of the toxins released get totally out of the body. A clear example is when mercury is dumped into the large intestine for passage out of the body. If a person does not have optimum passage time (18 hours from eating to bowel movement), they run the risk of reabsorbing the mercury. After the body does all that work to get the mercury out, it is right back in. An easy way to tell your passage time is to eat corn which passes virtually unchanged.

It is critical for patients to have bowel regularity before they begin getting metals out. The best way to do this is by increasing fiber from fruits and vegetables. Adding supplemental fiber is also valuable plus it is quick and fast. A good source is oat bran is available in health food stores. Adding a few grams of bran to meals can make a major difference. Trial and error is the best way to do it. Drinking enough fluids is also important to help build bulk. For women, this might be more difficult. Many women have chronic problems with normal bowel movements and many have taken laxatives for years; one of the best and safest is cascara sagrada, available at health food stores.

The amount of fiber recommended daily is about 30 grams, about one ounce, but most Americans get around 20. It is estimated that the caveman's diet contained 100 grams of fiber. Our bodies are still genetically the same as those of the caveman, so it may be that 30 grams are not enough. We eat one half pound (eight ounces) to three-quarters of a pound (twelve ounces) of food per day. You should try to eat high-fiber foods and take some supplemental fiber. Thirty grams should be the minimum goal. More is better. An added benefit is fiber does not contain calories.

Whatever the cause, it is important that it is corrected or it may be impossible to get the desired results from metal removal. If regularity is a problem and you cannot correct it, seek help before seeing the dentist. Try various methods until you have at least one daily bowel movement.

Many people experience the opposite problem, too many bowel movements, known as "Irritable Bowel Syndrome." Another form is Chron's Disease. Mercury could be the trigger in both diseases. Mercury has many ways to cause such problems, including encouraging yeast infections. Most people with these conditions are adept in handling them. In our culture there are stigmas around bathroom activities so we do tend to keep quiet about any problems.

Many people who seek metal removal are knowledgeable about their bodies. They can find what works best for themselves. Since you are interested, you should do your own research and follow a program you can handle. Read, ask, and experiment.

A new book by Dr. Hal Huggins and Thomas E. Levy, *Informed Consent*, discusses the problems they have found detoxifying patients. A vitamin or mineral that helps one person or most people can cause a negative reaction in others. One brand may work better than another. The more toxins you get out of your system, the more sensitive you can become if you are re-exposed. People react individually, so you have to be your own expert.

Following is a list of some over-the-counter detoxifiers: vitamin C (helps almost everyone but how much is the question), B vitamins, sulfur-containing amino acids like cysteine and glutathione, and the chlorophyll-containing chlorella, spirulina, and blue-green algae.

The use of thiotic (lipoic) acid is also highly recommended by practitioners. It is the main detoxer used in Canada, and is a free-radical scavenger.

It has taken decades for you to accumulate all the toxic overloads. It will take years to get rid of even part of the toxins. The point is that once you stop putting more toxins in, your body will go about righting itself. From that point on your toxin load will diminish. The rate at which your body will do its best is guided by its innate healing ability rather than some external attempt to accelerate the process. Sometimes slow is better than fast. Let how you feel be your guide.

Detoxing The Brain

Getting mercury out of the brain may take much longer. Mercury's half-life in the brain may be 10 or more years. In other words, in 10 years, only half of the mercury will be gone. In another 10 years, half of the remaining half will be gone, or 75 percent of the original amount. It may not be possible for all the mercury to leave the brain in a lifetime. Fortunately, once toxins are stopped from being added, the problems they cause should begin to reverse as healing begins. It is not necessary to get all the mercury out of the tissues before an improvement can be felt.

The body has ways to detox itself, but they are slow. The patient can help the detoxing process by eating nutritiously and maintaining good elimination through regular bowel movements and adequate urination, which are major exit routes for toxins. (Slow elimination gives time for toxins to be reabsorbed.) Sweating is another way to eliminate mecury and other toxins.

Vitamin C

Vitamin C is quite effective in detoxing the body. The current way to refer to this vitamin is as an "antioxidant" or a "free radical scavenger," because it neutralizes free radicals remaining from chemical reactions or from external pollution. That is why vitamin C is so effective against damage from smoking.

An adequate intake of vitamin C is especially important because it is involved in so many metabolic systems. While there may be different amounts recommended, it is hard to go wrong taking 1 to 3 grams a day. The late Dr. Linus Pauling, twice honored with rare, individual Nobel Prizes, recommended six grams or more on a daily basis for everyone.

Vitamin C is so effective that it will also neutralize the anesthetics used to numb the teeth and gums, because they are free radicals. For example, if a patient is taking a 1000 milligrams (mg) or more per day, as is commonly recommended, it may neutralize the anesthetic, making it difficult or impossible for the person's mouth to get numb enough to do fillings. It is recommended that you taper down to 1000 mg or less prior to treatment. Then the day before treatment and the morning before treatment, do not take any vitamin C. Right after treatment, it is a good practice to take 1000 mg. Repeat this pattern for each appointment.

If you are having appointments two days in a row, it should be all right to take the 1000 mg right after treatment the first day to help protect yourself from the mercury released during the treatment. It is also helpful to take a charcoal tablet just before treatment to absorb any mercury that gets into your stomach. However, avoid using charcoal routinely because it is so efficient, it absorbs needed minerals as well as toxic ones.

Other Means

In addition, the use of saunas may help sweat out toxins, even though they can make people feel weak as the toxins are driven out. An alternative to saunas is moderate exercise. In either case, know your limits. The way back to better health will take time. Do not push too hard and try not to get discouraged.

There are also certain chemicals and prescription drugs that increase the rate of detoxification. Recommending such procedures is one of those gray areas where the dentist can be considered to be close to practicing medicine. It seems logical that if mercury was put into a patient's body by dental work, it should be the responsibility of the dental profession to get it out. However, many mercury-free dentists are reluctant to advise their patients on these ways to speed up the elimination of toxins.

Some mercury-free dentists recommend special IV solutions to aid in detoxing. Some dentists work with physicians who will give these IV solutions before, during and after the removal of the offending dental materials. It is difficult to give guidelines for so many different recommendations. Hopefully, in the near future there will be a method of increasing the rate of detoxification acceptable as a standard of care.

Unfortunately, most physicians do not know much about the materials dentists' use or how to get them out of a patient. They do not have much interest in learning about this problem, either, because they have enough trouble keeping up with all the information on things they routinely treat. They do not realize the negative impact dental materials and procedures have on their patient's overall health. Their attitude might well be, "Dentists caused the problems, dentists should clean them up." The use of drugs and IV's to detox dental materials will be a source of debate for some time to come.

Detoxing Naturally

There are other reasons to be cautious. When these toxins are pulled from tissues where they have been stored, they can become more active. A patient's symptoms may be aggravated during the detoxing period. For example, the prescription drugs (not yet in common use) that accelerate detoxing, may cause a lot of irritability. Is this period of increased symptoms worth the increased rate of detoxification? Seriously ill patients must be extremely cautious.

The best person to judge the effects of a detox program is the patient. If you speed up the process and begin to feel worse, you may want to slow down. The most important point is that the sources of the toxic metals are no longer in the mouth. Once they have been removed, the body will be able to begin getting rid of its stored metals on its own.

Your best option is to be self-informed, then listen to the dentist's recommendations, and then do what seems reasonable. The majority of people just need to get the dental materials out of their mouths to begin to get healthy. The sicker a person is, the more help they may need, but the less able they are to rush their recovery. It took years to build up the toxins; they cannot be removed in a week. Expect to spend a year or two to slowly detox. You should also expect the recovery to be bumpy with good times interspersed with some relapses.

7

ELECTRICITY IN YOUR MOUTH

When two different metals are placed in saliva, an electric current called a galvanic current is generated by the escape of metal ions into the saliva. First reported in the scientific literature over 100 years ago, the existence of this current is common knowledge among any science student and certainly among all dentists.

Most people with fillings can recall getting some aluminum foil in their mouth by mistake or touching a metal filling with a fork. The resulting mini-jolt is caused by a discharge of the built-up electricity created by the galvanic current. The memory of the jolt and the bad taste sticks with you. Many people have a constant metallic taste, which is accepted as normal. Once all the metals are removed ending the galvanic current, the metallic taste leaves, too.

While all dentists know about galvanic current, it is not taken as a serious problem but only an irrelevant phenomenon. However, the galvanic currents generated in the mouth can be quite strong, strong enough to sometimes cause small muscle bundles to contract or spasm. This movement is like the high school science experiment where a frog's leg is made to move using the electricity in a battery. Unfortunately, the battery is now in your mouth and the muscle contractions caused may create spasms in the small muscles that control the lower jaw, leading to a lot of discomfort, even pain. These spasms are so common that they may cause Temporal-Mandibular Disorder (TMD). Patients often have relief of TMD symptoms following removal of their metals.

In one interesting case a Swedish woman claimed she regained her eyesight after the removal of a tooth with a metal filling. Dentists may scoff at this claim because they do not believe removing a metal filling could have that effect. In truth, if the current was strong enough, it may have blocked the woman's optic nerve.

Other Effects

It has been shown in current research both here and in Europe that each tooth influences and is influenced by other parts of the body. The example of an infected wisdom tooth affecting the heart is well-documented. If a tooth is being weakened by an electric current, the other parts of the body associated with that tooth will also be negatively affected. Unfortunately, most of the problems galvanic currents could cause are beyond our ability to diagnose at this time. Little research is currently being done to learn more about these effects, but in the future, research may show that the galvanic current may be the most dangerous and damaging side effect of having metals in your mouth.

Types of Electrical Currents

There are two types of electrical charges, positive and negative. The current flows from negative to positive. Mercury fillings are generally negative and gold is generally positive, but the current flow varies greatly because so many different metals are involved and the body is so complex. In fact, there are five different metals in mercury fillings that no gold needs to be present to create these currents. In other words, currents can be generated between the different metals within one filling.

Electrical charges are created by the action of acids on metals. When acids attack mercury in fillings, a negative charge is created when mercury ions are released into the air and saliva. From there the ions can be absorbed into the body through the lungs or even directly into oral tissues. The negatively charge ions can also be attracted to positively charged metals, such as gold. Mercury will readily plate gold so that any gold that is in the mouth at the same time as mercury will have mercury ions on its surface.

Electrical current also accelerates the breakdown (oxidation or tarnishing) of the silver in the filling. The silver in mercury fillings tarnishes just as a silver tray will tarnish. The fillings keep tarnishing as long as they are in the mouth. If you look at a piece of a mercury filling that is from between the teeth, you will find that it is coal-black, while the tops of fillings stay polished because chewing wears away the surface layer. The particles that are worn away can also be picked up by the body.

One of the other electrical effects happens when a gold crown is placed over a mercury filling. This creates an internal current which can cause the tooth to decay. Remember, a healthy tooth does not decay. A tooth has to be weakened, and strong galvanic currents may be enough to do it.

Official Position

It is written in the dental school textbooks on dental materials that it is wrong to place mercury and gold so they are touching or opposite to each other, where they will touch while chewing. It is believed that this separation reduces the galvanic current. It is more advisable that mercury and gold never be placed in the mouth at the same time, touching or not, because saliva acts as a conductor between the metals wherever they are located. Yet the guideline against placing mercury and gold together does not seem to matter to most dentists, who routinely place gold and mercury together. Maybe they have forgotten this rule or just slept through the lecture in dental school!

In fact, it is common for dentists to "help" their patients by placing gold crowns over pieces of mercury fillings (about half of all crowns have old mercury fillings under them). This practice increases the current within the tooth and drives the metals into the body through the tooth, rather than out into the mouth. You must be very specific that you do NOT want any mercury left under a new crown. Your dentist must agree to follow your wishes. You can even ask to look; after all, it is your mouth. There is no valid reason to place a gold crown over mercury and it should NEVER be done.

Checking The Charges

When each filling is checked with a voltage meter, it shows a charge and a number, such as -5 or +7 millivolts. Dr. Hal Huggins believes that it is important to remove the most negatively charged fillings (most electrically negative quadrant) first because they are releasing the most mercury. Practically, fillings are usually done by quadrants or quarters of the mouth: upper right, upper left, lower right or lower left. (See Fig. 1.1 p. 8.) He then recommends the second most negative quadrant be done at the second appointment and so on.

Other anti-mercury dentists do not believe removing fillings in order of their electrical charges to be important; that does not mean it is not important or that removing them in sequence is not critical. Since the dentist must start somewhere and since it may be very important, he may as well do them in sequence to be on the safe side. The exception is when there is an emergency or pain, which should be dealt with first.

Dentists who do not remove the fillings by following the electrical sequence usually begin with what they believe is the most obvious dental problem. Unfortunately, what that means to many dentists is that they first do the procedure that will yield the highest revenue.

"My Dentist Doesn't Check The Charges"

What should you as a patient do if the dentist does not want to follow the sequence when he removes your fillings? It is your mouth and body, so you have the right to be on the safe side. If your dentist does not have a meter that can measure the electrical charges, ask him if he could get one as other patients will need it done, also. If he refuses, you still have the right to seek treatment elsewhere.

Complete Removal

When you do have your metals removed, it is important that all the metal is removed. Any metal left can generate galvanic currents. It is not uncommon to see the smaller fillings generating the largest charges. It is also not uncommon for pieces of mercury filling material to be left when a new composite filling is done. Sometimes the mercury is left because it is hard to see, which is why it is important for dentists to use magnifying lenses when they check the teeth prior to placing the filling.

It is important that no amount of metal be left, no matter how small. Dentists who have supposedly removed all the mercury from a patient's teeth have been known to leave behind pieces of the old filling, from tiny specks to fairly large hunks. Out is out! All mercury must go before refilling. A speck smaller than a period may cause problems in sensitive people. Because these specks of mercury can be elusive, the removal process must be thorough. Unfortunately, pieces can also be left because of sloppy or rushed work. Personnel in a fast-paced, busy dental office may not be as thorough as you need them to be.

Once any other metal is placed, such as a gold crown, it is impossible to tell if any metals were left beneath it. X-rays do not penetrate metal crowns. (Before you agree to have any crowns done, remember that any metal, no matter what kind or how pure, may cause problems.)

Sequence of Replacement

It is common for patients having their mercury replaced with gold inlays and crowns to have the work done one quadrant at a time, but it is crucial to remove ALL the mercury fillings before the placing of the first gold restorations. Remember that the new, positively charged gold attracts the old, negatively charged mercury. The instant the gold is placed in the mouth, mercury will begin to contaminate it. What was to be nontoxic gold is "instantly" ruined.

Removing all the mercury fillings before any gold replacements are placed is not difficult to do: requires no extra appointments but must be properly planned. If you decide you want gold in your mouth, be sure the dentist has removed all the mercury before he cements any of the new gold dental work.

High Copper Alloys

A new form of mercury filling material called "high copper amalgam (mercury filling)" was introduced 20 years ago. The additional copper changes some of the poor physical characteristics of the old mercury filling materials. Unfortunately, the extra copper makes high copper amalgam more electrically active. The increased galvanic current increases the amount of mercury that can be released into the filling. (It has been suggested by one leading mercury-free dentist that the increase in multiple sclerosis patients—and its coming at earlier ages—is due to this change in the composition of mercury filling material.)

Dramatic Improvement

Every mercury-free dentist has had some patients who experience dramatic and rapid improvements in their health after removing their dental metals. Some "overnight" recoveries cannot be due to just the removal of the mercury, as pointed out by critics of the "60 Minutes" report on mercury fillings. It is true that the mercury cannot get out of the body that quickly and that the blood levels usually increase immediately after removal. Those result do not mean that the removal of the mercury fillings was not the reason for the recoveries. The recovery could have been due to the end of the electric currents that had been created by the mercury fillings. If it were you that had recovered, would you care about which reason as long as you got better?

Although these electric charges are strong and can cause many problems themselves, they are almost totally ignored or viewed only as a curiosity by the ADA and government agencies. Stories of people hearing radio stations through their fillings have been told for years. If these stories are true, they should be studied in depth. What physical mechanisms are involved and what is their effect on the nervous system? Are microwaves involved? There is much to learn about the effects of galvanic currents. The negative attitude of most dentists means that real investigation will not happen any time soon. Not much research has been done and little interest is shown, particularly in America. Hopefully, the truth will slowly come out through research in other countries.

8

WHAT ARE THE RISKS?

Risks Versus Benefits Analysis

"Risks versus benefits analysis" might sound like a boring subject, best left to accountants and insurance companies, but it is exactly how we make all our decisions. A good example is smoking. Twenty-five percent of adult Americans still smoke even though the risks are well-known. Each smoker has balanced the risks versus benefits and made a choice.

If a smoker is faced with a new situation, the balance may change, causing him to reevaluate his behavior, to rethink his risk versus benefits analysis. For instance, if a smoker's friends become nonsmokers, or his office stops allowing smoking at work, or his baby develops breathing problems, then the risks increase and it becomes easier to quit because the balance has changed.

We use risks versus benefits analysis when we decide whether to have a drink and then drive, or when we decide whether to drive at 55 mph or 65 mph, or when we decide to have French fries instead of broccoli. We use risks versus benefits analysis when we decide virtually everything we do.

As children, our parents decided what risks were acceptable for us to take. As we became more and more independent, we tried riskier things, usually with certain benefits in mind. Still, in some aspects of our lives we continue to let others make judgments for us. We may let religious leaders tell us what behaviors to follow because we believe that since they have studied theology, they have a better grasp of moral behavior. We may let a physician decide what medicine we should take because that is what he has studied. We may let a dentist determine what material to use for a filling without much thought. After all, these people should know their field and we are too busy to learn about it.

Maintaining Our Rights

> *Doctors should speak firmly to patients because it causes them to respect you and increases the size of your fee.*
>
> Unknown

We tend to give up our rights too easily. We are taught to accept certain people's judgments above our own, not because they are never wrong, but because we believe that they are acting first and foremost in our best interests. In addition, we come to believe that we cannot really understand their areas, and that others are much better-educated than we and maybe even smarter.

Our believing the professionals without question makes their lives much easier. Some professionals do not like their patients or clients to "think" because not everything they do can stand up to questioning. These professionals prefer people who "do as the doctor says," without having to spend their time justifying what they do. Loren Shahin, an accountant, often said, "People who think cause trouble." This observation contains more than a kernel of truth.

Blind faith may be a great idea in a perfect world. Unfortunately, we do not live in a perfect world.

The purpose of this book is to show the real risks versus benefits of dental procedures, so that you can make an informed decision and not be at the mercy of a dentist whose reasons may not be based on your best interests. It is entirely possible that a dentist may not even be aware of all the risks of a procedure. He may have done it so many times that he forgets to look at the risks versus benefits for each patient.

At least one person in every family should learn what is in this book. It is not required to learn all about dentistry or even technical aspects of treatments. But it is necessary to learn the general concepts underlying dental treatment so you can better evaluate what are acceptable risks. Many of these concepts are considered "inside" information. Knowing them will allow you to be aware of bad treatments and good treatments badly done, so you may protect yourself. The effects of many treatments can be so serious as to ruin your life.

The "Bionic" Mouth

In a country where we have been raised on "The Bionic Woman" and "The Six Million Dollar Man," it seems natural to believe that doctors can fix anything. Artificial hearts, hip replacements, and re-constructive surgery make the placement of a simple tooth implant seem like kid's stuff. The problem is there is no such thing as a bionic woman or six million dollar man; they are science fiction TV shows. An artificial heart that functions as well as a healthy heart will never be achieved. Hip replacements are common but no panacea. Reconstructive surgery does sometimes produce miracles but at an enormously high price both in money and potential trauma for the patient. Likewise, tooth implants are not simple or without problems. The longevity of the implants is a major factor, with failures marking every turn. The question is not, "What to do IF they fail?" but "What to do WHEN they fail?"

Mechanistic Concept of Dentistry

At the first commencement of the Harvard School of Dentistry (1872) Oliver Wendel Holmes warned about ". . . the danger of dentistry based upon a mechanical rather than a biological concept..."

This idea of replacing parts of a human being as if the body were a machine is a "mechanistic" concept of dentistry. But the body is a complex biological and physiological being that does not respond well when it is treated as if its parts were interchangeable. When patients are viewed from a biological, rather than a mechanical, point of view, a much greater need exists to place our emphasis on prevention of problems rather than on engineering re-placement parts. But as long as dentists continue to think that fixing things mechanically is the way to practice, there is no reason to prevent oral structures from being damaged. We think, "Why worry? When the natural structures break down, artificial ones can be made (for a price!)"

However, we are not machines. If we lose a part of our body, whatever we replace it with is NEVER better, and usually far worse, than the original. Not even the best artificial arm will make an amputee a major league pitcher.

Dental Training

The profession of dentistry has been trained to help you mechanically replace mouthparts that should never need replacing. If a person is missing a tooth, a bridge replacing will not function as naturally as the original tooth. It seems that we may not have cared a bit for the original tooth but once we have lost it, we are willing to spend a month's pay to replace it! Our parts are not really replaceable, and we need to treat the originals better and not rely on patches to make things work.

The problem is that professionals make no money in prevention, but the money comes from the repair after the damage has been done. Our professionals stand ready to help in every way they can, but only after the damage is done. In this sense the professionals are like predators, preying on the injured. Lawyers, physicians, and dentists all wait till we fall, then run in to put "Humpty Dumpty" back together again. While our bodies have some regenerative ability, we still need to value our "wholeness" more. We are far too willing to wait until we fall off the wall and shatter (become ill) before becoming serious about our health. Trying to regain lost health is a difficult quest, which is rarely fully successful.

It is most important that we attempt to keep the young people in good condition to prevent the problems now faced by adults. Then we can turn our attention to patching up the adults; unfortunately, we are not doing this. Our attention and money, both personal and governmental, are spent on correcting problems, not preventing them from happening in the first place.

Recommendation: Practice good health habits so you do not develop problems that need solutions. A CAVITY THAT DOES NOT FORM DOES NOT NEED A FILLING.

That's Good Enough

In any human endeavor, the quality of work is determined by the person's level of what is "good enough." This is the level at which each individual's standards are set. How often have you used that statement? You remember something you need to do, you are in a hurry, people are pressuring you. Finally, you stop working and say, "That's good enough!"

The pursuit of excellence has become the goal for many companies. For example, this pursuit is the "hallmark" of Hallmark, Inc., from the company's greeting cards to the TV shows it sponsors. Unfortunately, this pursuit has not been adopted by dentists when it comes to their choice of materials or procedures. And it is just not "good enough" to do a perfect filling with a toxic material.

Many factors determine how high a standard is used to judge dental work; one is your dentist's level of "good enough." Is his work the best he is capable of doing? Or is he being pressured to hurry and settle for less? How good is his best in the best of circumstances? Maybe he tries very hard but cannot equal someone else's average work. Remember, in every profession half of the practitioners graduated in the bottom half of their class. Or maybe they were once the best but now have lost some skill because they have acquired micro-tremors in their hands from mercury poisoning. Other problems can lower skill levels, such as substance abuse, emotional stress and time pressures.

Many people want to do better but are stopped by lack of talent. Not everyone wins the gold medal, no matter how hard they try and some dentists are just better than others. Still others do not even know their limits, so they do procedures that often end in disaster for their patients.

Skill Level of Dentists

Unfortunately, patients have little ability to tell one dentist from another. Many believe that all dentists are basically the same, performing procedures equally well. If you think about that belief for a few seconds, you will realize how wrong it is. Patients who believe they can go to a big clinic, staffed with dentists recently graduated from dental school, and still get quality care at rock-bottom prices are deluding themselves.

The generally accepted criteria do not apply. The most popular dentist, the busiest dentist, or the most expensive dentist may or may not be the best dentist. Finding a dentist that has high standards combined with an understanding of nontoxic materials and minimally damaging procedures is difficult. It is common to hear patients say that they are looking for someone to replace their mercury fillings because their last dentist would not do it or he would do it, warning that the white fillings "just wouldn't hold up." The patients then add, "But he's so nice." The question is not which dentist is nicest but which is using the least damaging procedures and materials in a most competent manner. In addition, he should attempt to prevent future problems by encouraging the patient toward better habits of diet and nutrition.

Competency of Dentists

Few dentists see dental work they would compliment. They routinely see dental work that should be replaced, not because it is worn out, but because it is poorly done. For every one percent of dentists who cannot do decent or better work translates into 1,500 dentists. How high is the number of incompetent dentists? As a general rule it is estimated that five percent of any profession, be it mechanics or brain surgeons, are too incompetent to practice their profession. To apply that percentage to dentistry means 7,500 dentists, or one out of 20, but that number may be too low. Is your dentist one of those 7,500 dentists?

The ability of many dentists to perform the types of work expected of a practicing dentist has been called into question by virtually every author and group including the ADA. Many critics make statements such as, the procedure is too "technique sensitive." Others come right out and say it. The author of *Dentistry and Its Victims* stated that 30 percent of dentists do not even care about the quality of the work they do and only 5 percent can do good-quality work. Is your dentist in the top 5 percent?

These are stinging indictments of the dental profession. If dentists are this inept, there should be mandatory retraining programs, not just a sloughing off of the problem by telling dentists to use the easiest materials, no matter if they are toxic or not.

Not Spreading The Word

One patient returned after five years to have some minor work done. She mentioned how her hives cleared up immediately after her nickel bridge was removed. She said the bridge was placed by a friend who was a dentist. This dentist friend attended her wedding and she still never mentioned that the nickel bridge caused her to have hives. She did not want her friend to feel bad. "How can this dentist learn that dental materials are a problem?" I asked. The patient shrugged. The social situation exceeded the truth once again.

Fair Compensation

Another reason why so much dental work is of low quality is because dentists are not well-compensated for routine fillings. Even if they wanted to switch from mercury to composite fillings, their experience tells them they will net less money from a composite filling. But even the mercury fillings are not compensated at a high enough rate to give the dentists the time needed to do the best they can do. And now, with the new pressure to control costs through managed care, the economic pressures will be worse.

Low compensation also puts pressure on dentists to push patients into more expensive procedures, such as inlays and crowns. Dentists are constantly told to promote "the finest dentistry has to offer," which usually means crowns. Patients and their teeth would be better off if dentists could earn the same rate, or even more, by doing the most conservative procedures rather than the most complex ones.

The real problem is that the profession is out of balance both in its leaders' attitude toward toxic metals in the dental material and the public's attitude of paying a fair price for good work. Currently, the leadership's collective heads are in the sand and people want something for nothing. As individuals, we do not have to tolerate these attitudes. We can take good care of our teeth and find a dentist who will take the time to do excellent work.

Personal Responsibility

Another reason, and one of the most important, is that a large percentage of our population does not take good care of their mouths. Even if the best quality of non-toxic materials are used with the best techniques, if a patient continues to sip sugared drinks throughout the day, nothing will work. In patients with good nutritional habits and who spend a reasonable amount of time in daily cleaning, dental work lasts indefinitely. In fact, even poor dental work will last a long time.

Quality of Dental Materials

Even the work of a dentist with excellent skills can be compromised by how he views the various dental materials and procedures. A dentist may think, "Mercury fillings may cause some problems but they're 'good enough' for my patients." Or "Nickel crowns may cause cancer in lab rats but they're 'good enough' for my patients!" Or "Root-canals may cause some immune system suppression but they're 'good enough' for my patients." A technically excellent dentist with an engaging

178

personality may put in a perfect nickel crown on a root-canal-treated tooth, but is that procedure in a patient's best interest? A combination of technical skill, good techniques, and biocompatible materials is what a patient should seek. If the dentist with these attributes also has a great personality, that is a bonus, but go for competence first.

What is "good enough" for you and your children? What kind of dentist do you want doing your work? What materials are "good enough" to use in your mouth? You need to answer these questions. The length and quality of your life may depend on the answers.

The Longevity of Dental Work

When we make the decision to buy a coat, we do not expect the garment to last the rest of our lives. Even with such an expectation, we would probably tire of the coat or it would go out of style, or our bodies would change and it would no longer fit. We are generally happy if we get a couple of seasons of hard wear out of a coat. We expect a bit more from of our cars and even more from our houses. But what about our teeth? We are very blasé about them, taking them for granted. We abuse our teeth so much that they actually rot in our mouths, and then we have them repaired with toxic materials about which we know nothing. With our little dental knowledge, we tell the dentist, "You're the doctor. Do what you think is best."

If we need a filling, we have it put in and do not worry about it until we need another one done. If we have a procedure done that is more expensive than a filling, we may ask about its durability, but we are much more likely to only ask about its cost.

When the dentist tells us it will last 10 or 15 years, we are satisfied because we can barely think ahead to next week. While 10 to 15 years sounds like a long time, it really is not compared to our life span. Almost everyone who reads this book has 20-50 more years left to live. If it is your last 20 years, the average filling on average will not last the rest of your life. Since most dental work will not last as long as the patient lives, additional work will have to be done when the original work fails.

Replacing Dental Work

Each complete replacement of a previous repair is always more difficult, and the more elaborate the previous procedure was, the harder it will be to replace it. If the previous procedure was too damaging to the tooth (all dental procedures cause some to a lot of damage to the natural tooth), there may not be another treatment possibility when it is time to replace it. Teeth get used up by wear, decay, gum disease, and yes, even DENTAL TREATMENT! To get teeth to last a lifetime, the damage done by any of these factors must be kept to a minimum. Therefore, the patient's general health, nutrition, and cleaning habits are critical to maintaining the teeth. Secondarily, not having bad habits such as tobacco use is very important.

Even after dental work is done, if the patient eliminates the condition that caused the problem, the dental work can last much longer. That burden is on the patient's shoulders. The need for a dentist's services must be kept to a minimum. The fewer repairs your teeth need, the more likely you are to keep them. Remember, if a tooth never has a cavity, it will never need the first filling. Without a first filling, it will never need a second one.

"How Long Will It Last?"

"How long will it last?" is a question that patients often ask when considering replacing their metal fillings with composites--a valid question, but one not usually asked of a dentist who is placing toxic metal fillings! Most dentists would answer that non-metal fillings do not last as long as metal ones. This is a half-truth. What they are really saying is, "I don't know how to make composite fillings that last as long as my mercury fillings." It is often not the material but the dentist's technique that is at fault.

No one challenges the fact that composites are more technically difficult to do, but why is it the ADA's major excuse in dismissing their general use? When dental students are first taught how to do mercury fillings, they find the procedure difficult, but they learn how to do it through practice. Currently, dental students must learn both mercury and composite filling techniques. If mercury fillings were no longer used, students would only have to learn one technique, so the training would actually be easier.

But what if the ADA is right and composite fillings are more likely to need replacing sooner than mercury fillings? Is the risk of an early failure more a threat to a patient's health than the presence of mercury in the body? Obviously, having a toxin implanted in your body would seem like a much greater risk.

Dr. Gordon Christensen

Dr. Gordon Christensen, a popular contributor to the ADA publications, wrote in 1989 in his Clinical Research Associates (CRA) Newsletter, that not only are composites and mercury fillings comparable in their life span, but mercury is by far the more toxic filling material. Overall, he rated the composites

181

higher! Four years later, in the May 1993 *Journal of the American Dental Association* (JADA), Dr. Christensen stated that composites "serve acceptably when compared to amalgam [mercury filling material], but patients need to know about them... "More people than you think have true allergies or sensitivities to metal." Now, since this was written in its own journal, the ADA can neither deny that there are problems with mercury nor that good substitutes are available. Unfortunately, Dr. Christensen states his opinion in such a way that dentists are not required to take action or to change their ways of practicing. The ADA may tolerate his statements because he does not call for an end to the use of mercury.

Attitudes of Insurance Companies

Insurance companies, because they face the potentially higher costs, are not in favor of changing all mercury fillings to composites. But they are looking at it from a monetary point of view, and you must consider it from a health perspective. It may be short-sighted of them to not see the greater health implications that follow the implanting of the toxic mercury in human bodies, but they should not be expected to lead the fight against the use of mercury; that should be done by dentists. Unfortunately, most dentists have failed to act in their patients' best interest, so the only ones left are the patients themselves. Therefore, it is up to us individually to protect ourselves and our loved ones.

Average Longevity of Fillings

While insurance policies generally will pay to replace a mercury filling after only one year of use, you should expect eight to ten years of use out of either material, depending on the skill used in placing them and the health of your mouth. But the longevity of the filling is not the real issue, and you should not be tricked into missing the point. Everyone wants the materials to last indefinitely. If the current composite materials do not last as long as we would like, new materials will be available before the replacement composites wear out that will last much longer. The ADA projection that these fillings will need replacement every 10 years or so for the rest of your life is based on current materials and techniques. It is probable that within 10 years, new non-metal materials will be introduced that will last much longer. If you want to wait until the perfect material is invented, it is your choice, but remember that mercury will continue to build up in your body until you get the mercury fillings out.

Other Factors

Besides the material itself, other key factors will determine how long a filling will last, including the thoroughness of your oral hygiene, your diet, and the skill of your dentist. If all are excellent, then you should expect your new composite fillings to last quite a long time. If the quality of any or all of these factors is poor, then even tooth enamel, nature's best material, can break down. If the factors that caused the original cavity are still present, then any filling material used will be under constant attack and its longevity will be shortened.

"What Happens Next?"

The idea of asking, "What happens next?" may be the most important concept you can get from reading this book, a concept that most patients, and dentists, do not consider when they choose a treatment option. Patients may ask, "How long will it last?" but they neglect to ask this next critical question, "What happens next?"

The reason this question is not asked is that dentists are taught to think mechanically. Viewing the mouth as a machine, they believe that if one part breaks down, they need only replace it with another. They think that this process can go on indefinitely, just as with a machine, that there will always be a way to fix it. But the mouth is not a machine; it is part of a living being and cannot be repaired by swapping a new part for an old one. A living organism can sometimes repair itself by healing, but a mechanical repair is not the same as healing.

"That's Not Biology, That's Engineering!"

When this wrong approach to dentistry was explained to a patient, he thought for a moment and said, "That's not biology, it's engineering!" That insightful comment sums up all the problems with the practice of dentistry. The comment could also point to a better future, if dentists begin treating people like living beings, instead of machines, if dentistry finally abandons its legacy of toxic materials and damaging treatments and becomes a true healing art.

Now, however, when a dentist sees a problem, he only thinks about how to fix it, giving little or no thought to its origin or how to prevent its recurrence. With dentists' reliance on mechanical repairs, is it any wonder that they are thought of as "tooth mechanics?" How do they spend their time with patients? At least 80 percent of their time is spent mechanically fixing teeth. As with our current approach to medical problems dentists attack the symptom and ignore the cause of the disease.

A Healthy Tooth Does Not Decay

Yes, it is true: A healthy tooth does not decay. A cavity is just a symptom of the tooth's natural self-healing ability being overwhelmed. Once a cavity forms, it does need repair, but the reason for the cavity forming in the first place should be found so future problems can be avoided. Remember, decay is 100 percent preventable. Decay can even be reversed without a filling if the natural healing can be restored. Dentists do not like that idea.

Recall the earlier example of a typical patient's treatment throughout their life: A small cavity becomes a filling at age 12. Eventually, more decay occurs, requiring a larger filling at 22, and then larger again at age 34. The next time the filling fails at 42, the dentist recommends a crown. In two years the tooth abscesses, necessitating a root-canal. At age 47, the tooth has become so damaged that it must be removed. At 48 a bridge is made, which fails by age 58 causing a partial denture to replace two teeth. Finally at age 65 the remaining teeth have become so weak that the patient needs the remaining teeth extracted and a complete denture. At each step the immediate problem, actually a symptom of an underlying problem was repaired mechanically. If a mechanistic approach is followed, then the continuing breakdown and inevitable loss of the teeth are predictable at age 12. That is not a healing art, but a "guided mechanical destruction of a living tissue."

The Real Answer Is Prevention

The second cavity should have never occurred. What would have stopped it? Sealants? Too late! Fluoride? If it could, but at what price to the rest of the body? Diet? Beyond the scope of dental practice. Dentists really do not have the training to answer the most important questions they face every day and therefore, continue to do only what they were trained to do, mechanically repair teeth. The causes of the diseases dentists treat are nutritional; therefore, the prevention of dental problems is tied to diet. But dentists are not trained in this area and are selected for dental school because of their skill with their hands not because they are interested in nutrition.

In fact, dentists are discouraged from treating patients nutritionally. In some states dentists are even banned from recommending vitamins and minerals. But even if they do advise their patients on nutrition, they are not compensated for such preventive services. Patients have been conditioned to expect dentists to merely fix the immediate problem, not tell them how to prevent it from happening again. They may even resent any nutritional questions a dentist might ask, mostly from the universal feeling that we do not eat right and do not want anyone to know. We may correctly feel ignorant or confused about what we should really be eating so we eat what we like and hope for the best.

More of the Same

"What happens next?" in most dental offices is usually more of the same or worse. You, as the owner of your mouth, must do the preventing. You must rely on yourself, or you may be one of the multitudes of our 65-year-olds with no teeth.

The damage you may do to yourself by poor food choices and bad habits is something you have to live with. The bigger damage done by well-meaning but short-sighted dentists is another matter altogether. Dentists are capable of turning a minor problem into a disaster. Let us assume you have caused a tooth that already had a large filling to have another cavity through poor diet and oral hygiene. Instead of rebuilding the tooth with a bonded composite filling or inlay, followed by improving your diet and cleaning habits, your dentist recommends a crown, a standard recommendation. The crowning procedure then causes the tooth to die (*The ADA News,* a semi-monthly newspaper for ADA members, reported there is a one in five chance of this occurring). That death leads to a root-canal, a possible apicoectomy (surgical removal through the bone of the end of the root) and maybe even the loss of the tooth. Is the loss of the tooth due to the cavity or the treatment choices made by the dentist? More importantly, how well-informed was the patient of the possible outcome of the treatments?

By asking, "What happens next?" you can avoid getting into treatment that requires increasing damage to be done. For example, if you know the probable next step after a crown is a root-canal, you are likely to avoid it by not having the crowning procedure done. You must stop dentists from doing unnecessary and irreversible damage to your teeth. All dental procedures must be kept to the minimum to limit the unavoidable damage they cause.

Remember the question "What happens next?" It will be a major help in guiding you to make the best decision when faced with difficult choices. You could also ask yourself that question the next time you buy a 32-ounce soft drink at the convenience store.

Governmental Attitude

Many federal government agencies try to point out dangers. For example, under Occupational Safety and Health Administration (OSHA) guidelines, every product used in a workplace is required to have a Material Safety and Data Sheet (MSDS), which states the various risks, including cancer and birth defects, associated with that product. The form must say what problems may be caused by short-term and long-term exposure. The current forms may be difficult to read but are being revised and made uniform. Hopefully, clearer and more readable forms will be available soon.

If you would like to see what the MSDS says about mercury, ask your dentist to show you his copy of the MSDS on mercury. If you do not understand it, the dentist can explain it to you. After you read the list of problems that mercury can cause, you may question why it is used in humans. It is up to you to decide if it seems like a material you want in your or your child's mouth. You may also wonder why your dentist did not inform you about these risks earlier, since this material is clearly not biocompatible.

Your dentist may believe that mercury is a hazard to only a few people and may deny ever having seen any problems in his patients. The reason he has not seen any problems is because he has not looked. Although the ADA acknowledges only 50 recorded reactions to mercury, many mercury-free dentists see hundreds a year. If depression is a common side effect of mercury, how many patients with depression does the average dentist see? Lots! But to find out if a patient has any of the symptoms listed as possibly caused by mercury, the dentist must ask and that is not done. Therefore, it is not surprising that dentists say they do not see mercury-caused problems.

Mercury is Toxic to Every Living Thing

The ADA speaks of "hypersensitivity" and "allergies" to mercury, but both terms are (perhaps intentionally) misleading. Mercury is toxic to every living thing; no level of mercury is considered safe. The levels at which individuals show signs of toxicity vary greatly, but the toxicity always increases with the amount of mercury, length of exposure, and strength of the immune system. One filling may severely damage a person in only a few cases, but even one mercury filling damages everyone at least a little. At what point will your mercury fillings damage you enough to lower the quality of your life? No one knows, but at some point mercury in the body is bound to exceed everyone's tolerance. Thus the ADA's insistence on describing mercury's damaging effects as "hypersensitivity" or "allergic reactions" is a gross understatement, but even these terms give some indication that mercury is not biocompatible. The ADA never uses the true terms: toxin or poison. Maybe they have not yet noticed the "skull and crossbones" symbol on the packages of mercury.

Another of the ADA's half-truths is that composites may be toxic. It is true that any man-made material is always less good for you than the natural material it replaces. And granted, while there may be some people who react to one brand of composite and not another, very few react to all composites. Those who do react may do so because their immune systems have been damaged by their mercury fillings. If the ADA is so concerned about patients reacting to any filling material, perhaps it should require compatibility tests before any fillings are done; that would give patients a clear indication of what materials they can tolerate. You can be sure that mercury will not be at the top of the list of compatible materials.

History of Routine Use of Composites

The part of the truth that seems to have been forgotten is that dentists have been routinely using composite materials for fillings in front teeth for 25 years. If dentists argue that composites may be as dangerous as mercury, why have they been using them in the front teeth for over two decades? And if composite and mercury are both dangerous, why are they using either? They cannot have it both ways.

Typically, the biocompatibility of composites has only been questioned because the ADA is trying the approach that the "best defense is a good offense." When mercury use is questioned, instead of answering, the question is ducked by focusing on potential imperfections of composites. However, pointing at the imperfections of other materials will not make mercury any less poisonous.

If the ADA persists in trying to take the heat off of mercury by portraying composites as just as bad, then the way to counter that argument is simple: Have an independent research group test every material for biocompatibility and compare the results. But before the ADA calls for a ten-year study, the comparisons have already been done by Dr. Gordon Christensen in his Clinical Research Associates (CRA) Newsletter. His comparisons showed that composites are superior to mercury fillings. Do not be misled by the arguments used against the replacements for mercury. The real issue is biocompatibility with your body.

The Philosophy of Dentistry

The underlying philosophy of all dental schools is the same: "Save every tooth." Sophisticated techniques have been developed to back up this philosophy. The problem is that these techniques are all mechanical repairs, based on the concept that the body is a machine; once its parts are replaced, it will be as good as new.

When this philosophy is taken to its logical conclusion, every mouth should be restored to its most complete level, using the finest and best mechanical techniques dentistry has to offer. This "Cadillac" concept of dental practice is embodied in the Pankey philosophy. Dr. Pankey, a true believer in the mechanical restoration of the teeth, taught that any damaged teeth should to be rebuilt with the strongest, best-looking and most functional materials available. Dentists trained at the Pankey Institute must take many courses over many years to be fully schooled in his techniques. His is the ultimate expression of the basic "save every tooth" philosophy.

But even dentists just out of dental school have been thoroughly indoctrinated in this dental philosophy. Each dental student is carefully led step-by-step into the basic philosophy during their four years of rigorous class work and clinical apprenticeship. This philosophy becomes so well ingrained by graduation that it can never be fully overcome. Even the most anti-mercury and anti-metal dentists will find that they still try to follow the basic philosophy. This blind following may account for the inability of the majority of dentists to challenge the validity of what they were taught, even if they come to realize that much of what they were so carefully taught is wrong.

Dentists' Attitudes Toward Mercury

The majority of dentists are not all that fond of mercury fillings and in time, will stop using them when a material without mercury is found that is as easy to handle. Dentists do not see using mercury as a "big deal." All drugs have a few side effects, so what if there are one or two people who react? Their belief is that if they ever see a patient react to mercury, they will gladly use something else, but never expect to see a patient who reacts.

On the surface this seems to be a reasonable viewpoint. Most dentists think that anti-mercury dentists are being foolish, like "Chicken Little" running around saying the "sky is falling." They have looked but see no problem. In fact, their biggest concern is that anti-mercury dentists are hurting the image of the dental profession. Actually, that much is true because as people learn the truth about dental materials, the image of dentists will suffer much more.

A New Dental Philosophy

The core of everything in this book is: NO TOOTH IS WORTH DAMAGING YOUR IMMUNE SYSTEM. This philosophy can never be fully compatible with the current dental philosophy because it does not view the body as a machine. This new philosophy takes a much broader view, recognizing that the mouth is part of the body and that whatever is done in the mouth has implications for every other cell in the body. Therefore, any material and technique has to be judged first by how it affects the whole being.

Intolerance to Inorganic Materials

We live and die on the cellular level
Ted Moeter, Jr., D.C.
Author and Past President of Logan College of Chiropractic

No pure metals are known with which living tissues are fully compatible. True, some metals can be tolerated, and if there is a real need, the risk may be worth it. For example, if you cannot walk because of a damaged hip that can be replaced with a titanium joint, you have a need worth the risk. But if you have a decayed tooth, what risk are you willing to take to have a filling? What if a more biocompatible material had one-tenth the risk at only a 25 percent increase in cost? Maybe you think it would be a

193

good trade-off, but your insurance company or PPO clinic wants you to use the cheaper one. Whose interests are they protecting? If a filling material makes it difficult for you to think, is it a bargain at any price? Or if saving a tooth with a root-canal causes you liver damage, do you really want to save it?

If there is any question about what material or technique to use, the patient should at least have the option to be tested for any sensitivity with a compatibility test. As a patient, you also have the right to know about the side effects and to determine whether saving a few dollars or saving a tooth is worth risking your health.

The future of dentistry lies with this new philosophy. The question is not whether the philosophy will be implemented, but when it will be implemented--now or in fifty years. If the ADA has its way, this new and sensible philosophy will be slowly integrated into the profession, but that will take too long for every person whose health is now being destroyed by the use of toxic, non-biocompatible materials.

A Call For The Creation of a New Standard of Dental Care

Dentists should know what makes a good or excellent dental material and, in addition, what techniques conserve the natural tooth structure. Why are dentists not using this knowledge to guide their current treatments? Could it be that dentists do not care? No, most are concerned about the welfare of their patients. Could it be that dentists make more money doing procedures that may be of questionable value? Yes, that is part of the problem because economics drives all professionals, and dentists are no exception. These economic pressures are also used by some dentists as a rationalization to over-treat. If the time and money being used to do unhealthy and unnecessary procedures were applied to replacing the toxic materials and infectious treatments of the past, then there would be more work to do than all the dentists could do in their lifetimes.

Technique Sensitivity

Another also the claim is that the new composite materials may be too "technique sensitive," that is, so difficult to use that many dentists cannot do them. It has been estimated that up to one-third of all dentists would not be able to do composites successfully, but that number may be too high. Many older dentists may not want to retrain themselves, but the vast majority of dentists should be able to master any and all of the techniques. The keys to doing a good composite filling are to keep the tooth dry and take the time necessary to do it right. Repetition and experience should be enough to form the new skills needed.

Tradition

Then what is stopping the vast majority of dentists from following the higher standards? The nicest word in answer would be "tradition." Dentists have been treating patients the same way for many years. The older dentists who train the new dentists use the ideas they were taught. A lot of minds must be changed that do not want to be changed. "If it ain't broke, don't fix it!" is a commonly expressed thought, and dentistry is no exception. Dentists may feel that things will change in their own good time and that there is no reason to rush to replace the old materials.

That outlook would be all right if 150 million or more people in America were not being affected by these materials. People who are troubled by lack of energy, daily headaches, and depression, to name a few of the problems that these toxic dental materials cause, may think differently. These people have a right to be better now, not in 50 years. They did not place these toxic materials and infectious treatments in their bodies; dentists did. A dentist's good intentions do not count if your life is ruined.

Ego Can Slow The Process

It has been said that "at every crossroad to the future, there are 10,000 men guarding the past." Ego may also play a large role in preventing dentists from admitting that what they have done in the past may have been less than perfect and that their patients may have suffered for it. History is full of examples of egos slowing progress. Medical history is full of examples of patients suffering because doctors were slow to accept or even bitterly opposed, new concepts. For example, it took decades to get doctors to wash their hands between patients, even after the connection between their contact and new infections was proven.

Dentists, likewise, tend to be conservative by nature. In fact, part of Dr. Pankey's philosophy of dentistry is that a dentist should not be the first to accept a new idea. Since not all new ideas are good ideas, he advised waiting until the idea was proven beyond doubt. He then added that they should also not be the last to accept the new idea. This Pankey idea has some validity. One does not want to follow a will-o-the-wisp, flitting here and there, following every new idea, with no real direction. But there is a difference between being the first to use a brand new technique

196

and resisting a concept that has been around a long time, is readily provable, but politically unpopular.

Maverick Dentists

Since so many dentists use the "save every tooth" philosophy as a guide, who, then, will advance the profession in the needed new direction? Only the independent or maverick dentists remain. Mavericks dentists who believe they see a better way to practice dentistry and have for over a decade advocated getting the mercury out of people's mouths are certainly not looked on fondly by the majority of dentists. But instead of attacking these dentists as heretics against the status quo, the dental majority should make them stand up and show what they have discovered. They should listen openly to the their results and try to duplicate these results with their own patients.

Unfortunately, this reaction does not happen. Instead, dentists who oppose the use of toxic materials have worked, mostly alone, developing new ways to help patients. Slowly, they have grown in numbers and become organized into groups. They have tried unsuccessfully to demonstrate to other dentists through scientific research the faults of the traditional dental methods and materials, but these dentists turn a deaf ear. At the same time the 1994 Mid-Winter Dental Convention was held in Chicago, an alternative materials seminar was held nearby. Any interested dentists, among the approximately 20,000 attending the big meeting, were openly invited to attend free of charge. About 100 dentists came, about five-tenths of one percent. After a decade of trying, the message is not getting through to the mainstream dentists.

If these mainstream dentists will not listen, let alone adopt these changes, then the patients must do it for themselves. It seems obvious now that it will take informed patients to force the profession to follow a more biological approach to treatment. Sometimes a profession can only be changed by those on the outside.

9

HOW ARE TEETH DAMAGED?

Dr. Weston Price

> *Life in all its fullness is Mother Nature obeyed.*
> Weston Price, D.D.S.

Dr. Weston Price was a highly respected research dentist who worked in the first 40 years of the 19th century. For several decades he was employed by the American Dental Association (ADA) as head of its research programs. Dr. Price's decade-long research on root-canal therapy resulted in two large volumes, *Dental Infections, Oral and Systemic* and *Dental Infection and The Degenerative Diseases*, which warned of the dangers of root-canals, because chronic bacterial infections and toxins are left in the tooth (see "Root-canals"). Unfortunately, his work has been largely forgotten or ignored by the dental establishment, but his conclusions have never been disproved.

After leaving his post at the ADA, he traveled the world. Taking photographs of native people in Polynesia and other remote areas, he was able to show the influence of the Western (American) diet on children in the same families raised before sugar and white flour were introduced and those born after its introduction. The children exposed to sugar and white flour had dental disease and their faces were narrower, causing bad bites with crowded, crooked teeth. In some places, when the Western diet stopped being available, children born after the previous native diet was resumed were again healthy, just as the older children and the parents. Dr. Price's book about his observations of dietary influences on growth and decay, *Nutrition and Physical Degeneration*, has become a classic in nutritional literature.

Another Researcher

A colleague of Dr. Price, Francis Pottenger, M.D., did dietary experiments, using cats. When fed Western diets (human foods), the kittens grew with all the health problems we exhibit including allergies and deformed dental arches. When these kittens became adults, he fed them their natural diet, and it took five generations before their kittens were completely healthy. When the experiments were extended by feeding the cats the Western diet for three generations, none of the kittens survived to breed.

These experiments suggest that after long exposure to the Western diets, the facial deformities common in America--the long, narrow faces with crowded, crooked teeth--will become more common and harder to correct, even if we return to proper eating habits. In America, we are on our third, fourth, or fifth generations raised on high-sugar and white flour diets. In 1880 the average person ate 10 pounds of sugar per year. We now average between 120 and 150 pounds per person per year. While some people consume less, many people eat much more, mostly young people. Eating so much sugar is a cause of many of our major health problems, including most dental problems, but this problem is all but ignored by health practitioners and our government. In fact the food industry claims that our high sugar consumption is not a problem but a benefit. While our food industry boasts about how well-fed Americans are, the truth is that we are "overfed and undernourished." Chronic health problems plague a large percentage of our population. From diabetes to obesity to crooked teeth, our American diet shapes our lives for the worse.

How We Eat

...in the mouth will be found evidence of more disease than in any other region of the body. Such changes will be in the form of nutritional changes and infections around the gums, teeth and the tonsils. "

C.H. Mayo, M.D. 1922

A burger, fries, and soft drink seem to be many Americans' idea of a balanced meal, but this idea is a fabrication of the fast food industry, not reality. We still have time to return to whole foods, such as fresh fruits and vegetables, before further damage occurs. These foods are readily available and cost less than the processed foods. Our concept of what is good to eat has to change, if we want our children to develop healthy bodies, but we have to be strong enough to resist the power of modern advertising.

The simple truth of Drs. Price and Pottenger's studies places them in opposition to the interests of the food industry. Power and influence are always with the money, and the food industry has the money. That means we, as individuals, must learn what good nutrition is and then practice what we have learned. This strategy can only succeed one person at a time because it is in our self-interest. Since food processors are businesses whose basic intent is to sell their product, they will produce better foods as we demand and buy them. But if we let the food processors choose for us, it will be their interests that are served, not ours.

Genetic Health

In the course of Dr. Price's research, he formulated a theory about human beings' genetic ability to resist disease, identifying three main groups of people. One group is composed of healthy people with strong genetic backgrounds of healthy ancestors. These people may abuse their health all their lives with little noticeable effect. You may have heard people talk about someone who smoked 10 cigars a day, drank a quart of vodka for breakfast, and ate food cooked in lard but who lived to be 97 and died in his sleep on his fourth honeymoon. Such a good genetic background is fortunate. If you are 60 and your parents are still alive, you probably have good genes. If you are sixty and both sets of your grandparents are still alive, your have a superb genetic background. Long life and good health are your birthright.

Dr. Price stated that these people are so healthy that their immune system could even tolerate root-canal treatment; that may be true, but it is also true that they are the least likely people to need one. They tend to have good or excellent teeth, with little or no decay. Such people are usually so healthy that they would not need to read this book.

At the opposite end of the spectrum are people who seem to be ill all the time, beginning at birth. They tend to be sickly as children. As adults, their list of health problems is long, and they spend a lot of their time seeing doctors, but do not get better. These people have family members who have similar health patterns and some may die young, maybe an uncle who died in his forties from a heart attack. They catch every cold or flu virus that comes along, using up all their sick days at work. They have had several surgeries for one thing or another and have had organs removed, like tonsils, gall bladders, uteri, and appendixes. They are likely to lose their teeth at an early age. People in these families tend to die in their sixties or earlier.

In the third group, between the two extremes, is where most of us belong. If we take good care of ourselves, we can live reasonably long, healthy lives. But when we abuse ourselves with poor nutrition, we end up with many health problems, including a mouth full of fillings; if they are mercury fillings, the problems can be just that much worse. We may find that health problems occur even when we take good care of ourselves, e.g., when we do not eat or drink to excess and do not smoke. We may exercise routinely, sleep well, have good jobs, and enjoy happy, fulfilling relationships. But we still get chronic health problems for no particular, or at least obvious, reason and no doctor can find an answer. Look to your mouth. These chronic health problems may not be caused by "bad genes" but by toxic dental work.

Types of Dental Patients

The types of dental patients also fall into three groups partially resulting from the three genetic groups discussed above: A small group with few if any problems who do not need to see a dentist very often; a larger group that has awful teeth that they lose when they are young; and the majority, who need continual visits to a dentist in the attempt to maintain their teeth.

People with the poorest health, those in the weakest genetic group, lose their teeth early in life. It is not uncommon for some of these people to have dentures before they are 30. Their dental problems are symptoms of deeper health problems. Poverty can play a role in bringing about these problems, but ignorance is the biggest problem. These people may have genetically weak teeth to begin with, but that may not be the most important factor. Dentists commonly see genetically weak teeth that survive a lifetime. So what is the most important factor? The person's mindset. Many patients believe they will end up wearing dentures because their parents have dentures. Not knowing any better, they see it as "natural" for them to lose their teeth. They may even neglect having any dental work done that would slow the loss of teeth because they see losing their teeth as a certainty. This outlook shows a belief in a fate over which they have no control.

Is tooth loss a certainty or is it genetic? It is quite possible that what people eat, not their genetics, determines their "fate." People tend to eat what they were fed as children, which are the types of foods their parents ate as children. The foods we prefer may go back for generations; that means it is not weak teeth that run in the family but poor eating habits.

Understanding a problem through hindsight is easy, but what about your children? You cannot do much about what you were fed as a child, but you can change what your children and grandchildren eat now. Although it may seem difficult at times, you can break the cycle. What we feed children today will create habits that will determine the health of our future generations. Good food means good health; poor food means poor health. Unfortunately for many Americans, we see the pattern Drs. Price and Pottenger wrote about 50 years ago. We are passing down our own health problems from generation to generation, and they are worsening in spite of all the new information that is being given to the public through the media as the results of new studies.

The idea of a poorly nourished pregnant woman giving birth to a weak child is not new. If that woman has several more children, with each birth she may be less able to give the developing infant all the nutrition it needs. In addition, this poor beginning is followed by a childhood of poor nutrition, and the children's health can only get worse. When the children mature and have babies of their own with no better nutrition than they had, the health problems compound. We can now see chronic deficiencies going on for generations.

Chronic Deficiencies

Chronic deficiencies may not be due to having too little money because it is not expensive to eat healthy. Fresh foods are often bargains. It is the junk foods and fast foods common in today's diets that are expensive, both in initial cost and future medical and dental treatments. For instance, people love French fries, even though they are fried in partially hydrogenated, rancid oils. Some French fries are even covered with sugar to give them a crispy coating that browns nicely. After being covered with salt, we dip them in catsup, which is about 30 percent sugar. We think they taste great, but are they healthy? Eaten once a month, they may be "no problem," but eaten several times a week, which is a more likely average, and they begin to have a negative impact on our health. And these fries are not much of a bargain--about a dollar for a single order. That same dollar could buy two or three pounds of potatoes at the supermarket, which would obviously make many more servings. It is not the potato that is at fault but what we do to it.

Remember, 100 percent of dental problems are preventable. If a mother had a good diet as she was growing, her children will have a better chance of having good bodies, including teeth. The opposite is also true. If the mother had a poor diet as she grew, the chances are her children will be born weaker, and they will learn to eat poorly as they grow. So it is not just a teenage girl's dental health that is at risk when she drinks six soft drinks a day, it is the dental health of her future children, too.

Negative Mindset

Patients commonly say to their dentists, "I want to keep my teeth," but then add, "as long as possible." Their mindset shows that the message that all dental problems are preventable is not understood. Most people are surprised when they do not have a new cavity at their checkups. They believe getting a cavity will happen to them no matter what they do, that it is not something they can prevent. Perhaps going to the dentist is like confession; you know you have been bad but you hope that God will be lenient by not punishing you with a new cavity.

People with no dental problems seldom go to the dentist. So the majority of patients who routinely visit dentists have a history of self-inflicted dental problems. The health of their teeth and gums tend to go downhill slowly at first. The loss of teeth accelerates in their 40's and 50's, when damage from habits catch up to them. Many of these people lose their teeth and get dentures before they are 60. But if they can make it to age 60 in reasonable dental health, they will probably be able to keep their teeth the rest of their lives.

How Sugar Affects The Teeth

In the 1950's a dental researcher, Dr. Ralph Steinman, demonstrated that fluids flow from inside the tooth outward to the mouth. At first it seems hard to believe that fluids can flow through enamel because it is so dense and hard, but remember, the tooth is a part of the body, so the enamel has some organic tissue in it. As the fluid flows through the tooth, it nourishes the dental tissues, repairs damage, and flushes out the bacteria.

However, this flow can be stopped and even reversed by the impact of high sugar levels, which suppress the hormone that regulates the fluid flow. Without the hormone the flow stops. Then the flow reverses, and fluids from the mouth begin to flow into the tooth. These fluids contain whatever is present in the mouth, most of which affects the tooth negatively. For example, bacteria within the plaque that commonly covers teeth (particularly in patients who eat enough sugar to cause this fluid reversal to happen) can move into the tooth rather than be flushed out.

Brushing Is Not Enough

It is common for patients who have just been told that they have several new cavities to protest because they brush several times a day with a fluoridated toothpaste. Usually, after a few questions concerning their sugar intake, particularly soft drinks, they begin to grudgingly accept responsibility. When asked if they floss, they usually admit that they are not doing as good a job cleaning as they thought. It is doubtful that they will decrease their soft drink consumption for very long, and statistics that show few people routinely floss. It seems to be surrender to the fate of having to have filings done as a penitence for their nutritional and cleaning "sins". One 40-year-old patient, who needed and wanted his teeth out, when asked about his soft drink habits said, "I could never give up my Mountain Dew for breakfast!" He was giving up his teeth instead.

Until Dr. Steinman published his studies 30 years ago, it was believed that if you got sugar on your teeth and did not clean it off, you would get cavities, a simple cause and effect relationship. In fact, the ADA still tells the public in its pamphlets that plaque on the teeth causes cavities by the plaque bacteria consuming the sugar, which causes acidic waste products. The ADA further says that this acid eats holes in the enamel which allows bacteria in, thus causing the cavity. What the ADA does not point out is the more complex internal process caused by the sugar. The decay process is complex but the cause is simple, high sugar consumption. Why would the ADA give people "incomplete" information? Why does it not proclaim loudly and constantly that we must limit sugar consumption? The association must know about Dr. Steinman's research, yet does not think people are smart enough to understand. Maybe, the ADA is afraid to admit being wrong, just as it is about mercury fillings.

Plaque Is Not To Blame

To be absolutely clear, please read the following statement carefully: PLAQUE ALONE DOES NOT CAUSE DECAY. While high levels of plaque play a role in the destruction of the tooth, it is not the cause, but merely a symptom, of the same problem, faulty nutrition. Plaque is only present in potentially damaging quantities when we eat the sugar that stimulates it to grow, really overgrow, like an over-fertilized lawn. Anyone who eats sugar will have plaque on their teeth, particularly at the edge by the gums and between the teeth, where there is little or no natural cleansing from "detergent" foods, such as apples. The truth is, if plaque alone were the cause of decay, no one would have any teeth left, because decay would occur everywhere beneath the plaque and stopping it would be impossible. Dentists see patients with plaque-covered teeth that do not have decay. They also see patients with clean teeth that have cavities. If plaque were the sole cause, the two examples above could not happen.

In Dr. Steinman's experiments he fed laboratory animals a high-sugar diet, but he did it by putting the sugar directly into their stomachs using feeding tubes. No sugar ever touched the animals' teeth. Nevertheless, they all got cavities. That experiments showed that the key effect of sugar takes place on the inside of your body. This internal process is the most important factor in the formation of decay.

No Official Change

Although Steinman's research was published before 1970, the ADA still has not adjusted its position. After three decades it seems time for the ADA to get the message and quit preaching the dogma of brushing, flossing, and fluoride as the key ways to prevent decay. If you stopped the sugar, then you could skip doing all three, which is what every human did until the modem era and they did not have to worry about decay. A natural diet and decay are not found together. Animals in the wild eat a natural diet. Do wolves brush their teeth? Or killer whales? Brushing, flossing, and fluoride treatments are not needed because they eat in harmony with their bodies. Only humans believe they can disobey nature and not suffer the consequences.

Must you to stop eating all sugar to prevent decay? In America, stopping would be virtually impossible because of all the hidden sugar in processed foods. But it is possible to greatly reduce the amount of sugar you consume without lowering your enjoyment of life. Discussing diet and nutrition with people is difficult. It has been said that it is easier to get people to change their religion than their diet. But a total change may not be required; just a modification, slowly improving the quality, can help a great deal. For example, if you are drinking four cans of pop a day, you could reduce your intake to two cans, then to one over several months, without really disrupting your lifestyle.

Changing too much or too fast will cause resistance even if it is yourself who wants the change. If a woman tells her family that she is going to improve all their diets by fixing only "healthy" foods, she will meet more resistance than she can handle. The secret is in slowly changing what and how we eat. Lead by example.

A dentist who seriously discusses diet with his patients is usually not appreciated and likely will not be compensated for nutritional consultation. Patients may expect to be told to cut back on the sugar and brush better, but they do not want lectures on how to eat. This attitude is partly due to their view of dentistry as a profession that repairs teeth, rather than as a source of nutritional information

Decay

Man is a creature of natural law, and he must follow it. The penalty for disobeying the laws of nature are poor health, degenerative diseases, and eventual extinction.

Melvin Page, DDS
Author of "Your Body Is Your Best Doctor"

Tooth decay has many names: The official name is "dental caries" and the popular name is "cavities," but patients will say, "I have a hole in my tooth" or "I have a black spot." Decay is the breakdown of the hard tissues of the tooth, the enamel and dentin, the result of bacteria successfully attacking the tooth. These bacteria turn the hard tissues soft as the calcium structure of the tooth is destroyed. The process can be fast moving or slow and happens at some locations more than others. More importantly, IT IS 100 PERCENT PREVENTABLE!

Shakespeare wrote, *"What's in a name? That which we call a rose by any other name would smell as sweet."* Would that hold true for "decay?" It would not statement seem so innocent if a dentist were to use some word other than decay, such as putrefy, spoil, decompose, disintegrate, crumble, or ROT. Consider the effect if the dentist said, "You have some rot in your tooth." "ROT? Like the spot on an apple I cut out before I eat it?" the patient might reply. Although it sounds blunt, "rot" is a much better word because over the years the term "decay" has lost its impact. When a tooth has "decay," we may not even use the word but substitute the even softer word "cavity." We need to grasp the reality of what has happened to us; our tooth is "rotting within our mouth!" If we can actually grasp the reality of what is happening

211

to us, we may be moved to take action to stop it from ever happening again. That is what a reasonable person would do; that is what we all should do.

Think of the impact of the statement that part of our body, actually the hardest two tissues of our body, are "rotting." "I'm alive but I've begun to rot?" should be the reaction. "Isn't that supposed to happen after I'm dead?" The truth is that once we die, the teeth last longer than any other part of the body. But while we are alive, many of us cannot keep our teeth healthy for 10 years.

Many people are pleased when at their check-up, the dentist only finds one tooth with decay. Maybe when a cavity is found there should be a reading of the definition of decay like the police read the "Miranda Rights" to someone they arrest. It might say,

You have the right to slowly ruin the health of your mouth, to decompose your enamel and cause your teeth to fall into a ruined state. If you choose to give up this right to abuse yourself, you may choose to improve your diet by giving up the right to excessively eat sugar. If you do not understand these rights, you may begin to learn through self-education.

We Tolerate Dental Decay

Another way to look at the seriousness of dental decay is to consider how we would react if decay happened elsewhere in the body. If you got up one morning and found decay in one of your

212

fingernails you would be very upset. You would phone a doctor immediately, trying to find out what you should do and wanting to know why such a thing could have happened. The doctor might ask if you had been soaking your nail in sugar water. Of course not, you would never do anything that would cause part of your body to rot.

Our acceptance of rot in our teeth is why we have a mouth full of toxic metals. If people did not tolerate decay, filled teeth would be a rarity. You might have one filling due to an accident, but not from being brainwashed by commercials for the "good life" found by eating and drinking sugar-laden foods. Fortunately, you still have time to act on this new way of looking at decay. You have the power to make "tooth rot" a thing of the your past. For the rest of the book the more conventional terms "decay" and "cavity" will be used, but whenever you see them, think ROT!

Requirements For Decay

Three things are required for decay to occur: A tooth, specific bacteria, and food for the bacteria to eat. The key bacteria are acquired from others when we are infants and are with us the rest of our lives. Therefore, it is not whether we have bacteria, because we all do, but it is the quantity that is important. These bacteria are not a threat to teeth when in small numbers but only when they begin to grow into huge colonies; for this to happen they must have specific foods namely sugars.

Since we all start with teeth and we all have the bacteria, clearly the only one of the three factors we can really change are the sugars on which they feed. The ADA does not look at it this way. In a "special supplement" to *the Journal of the American*

Dental Association in June 1995, the ADA gave "A Review of Preventative Strategies and Management" of dental caries (decay). Their approach is to intervene with the tooth through various fluoride uses and procedures, like sealants. They also have strategies to reduce the bacteria to low levels through cleaning techniques and chemical therapies. Only a bare mention of diet is made.

Fluoride and sealants are discussed in other areas but are basically techniques that can be done to protect people from themselves. The cleaning techniques and chemical therapies are ways to clean up a mess after it occurs. The real way to avoid decay is to avoid the very thing that you can control, if our sugar intake. A simple method to reduce the impact of sugars while not lowering the amount you eat is to eat it with other foods. Using only this one method lowers decay rates 75 percent. Not only do the bacteria have less time to digest the sugars in the mouth, the impact on the blood sugar levels is reduced as absorption is slowed.

The real way to reduce the impact of sugar is to reduce the total consumption with or without meals. Without high levels of sugar the decay-producing bacteria do not grow to population levels that are damaging. You will not have to clean layers of plaque off your teeth if you do not grow these layers in the first place. It may seem too simple but the truth is that our food choice is the problem. Altering these choice immediately changes our susceptibility to decay. Without constant food—sugars—the number of damaging bacteria will rapidly decline. If, on the other hand we wish to grow them, sipping on soft drinks is the best way. Unfortunately, many of us think that having a soft drink is a necessity of life.

Obscuring Their Viewpoint

It is disturbing that the ADA supplement can say many of the same things contained in this book but do so in such a way that the truth is obscured not illuminated. In addition, a disclaimer appears at the beginning to the supplement, "The views expressed in this supplement to *The Journal of the American Dental Association* do not necessarily reflect the opinions or official policies of the American Dental Association or its subsidiaries." If it comes from the ADA and is copyrighted by them, whose opinions and policies can it reflect?

The other critical statement that shows the mindset of dentistry is that decay should be treated as an infectious disease; this is clearly wrong. You can have huge amounts of these bacteria even if there are no teeth. All dentists have seen dentures covered with plaque. So the bacteria are present but no disease is going on because there are no teeth. If it is an infectious disease, then any person with such large numbers of bacteria would have it. It is not an infectious disease but a degenerative process brought about by the improper ingestion of manipulated foods.

If you eat corn, you will not decay your teeth. But if the corn is changed into corn syrup, it can. With corn syrup the sugar concentration is so high that it will feed the damaging bacteria and will alter the internal body chemistry. A continuing exposure to such foods will cause decay to occur.

The ADA supplement refers to the diet only nine times in 24 pages. The following six phrases are used:

patient behaviors,
nutritional counseling,
dietary counseling,
available foodstuff,

fermentable carbohydrates, and
behavioral factors.

These references are at best, vague. Would you know that what they are talking about is eating too much sugar? In fact, the word sugar is never mentioned in the text and only three times in special information boxes. In contrast, the word fluoride is used over 120 times, thus showing where the emphasis is placed. Dentists are trained to do treatment, not to modify behaviors.

Changing behaviors is not compensated or always appreciated. One Halloween the idea to give out fancy children's toothbrushes was tried to make a counterpoint to all the candy the children received. The children felt shortchanged, and some of the parents thought that it was a marketing ploy. The experiment was not repeated. Perhaps most dentists have tried changing their patients' behavior but have met with such resistance that they have decided it is not worth their efforts. More probable is that they accept what they see as normal in our society and do their work to repair the damage caused by our diet. Changing the American diet may be viewed as outside their area of influence. That is why, to some, backing water fluoridation seems like the best way to fight dental decay. Slip them a bit of "prescription medicine" in the municipal water supply and it is back to drillin', fillin', and billin'.

Osteoporosis

Women are constantly told that they are at risk for osteoporosis. The group at highest risk is postmenopausal white women but it affects many others, too. Many factors seem to act in local areas, as well as, systemically. Many of the risk factors are in what we eat and drink. Too much red meat causes calcium loss. Any carbonated soft drinks cause calcium loss which may be one of the biggest problems in America. Lack of exercise, smoking and fluoride also contribute to the problem.

Women are told that it is the decrease of estrogen at menopause that starts the loss; that is true, but taking estrogen replacement is not as good an answer as it is touted. Estrogen helps for a while but after a few years there is little or no benefit. If you are prescribed estrogen to protect your bones, ask a lot of questions so you know what the most recent research shows. Research reports change so often a final answer cannot be found in any book.

Soft drinks cause the loss of calcium. Those drinks have high levels of phosphates to keep them from being too acid. The body requires calcium to remove the excess phosphates. Americans drink an average of 54 gallons of soft drinks a year. That means a lot of calcium is lost. When this loss is discussed with patients they act as if you are against the American way of life. "What can I drink? Water?" Heavens no, we cannot expect people to drink water! Thankfully, many people are switching to water. We are willing to pay the same for water as we are for other drinks.

Red meat contains little calcium. The way we prepare our meat is one of the reasons. If the bones are thrown into the stew pot, calcium will get into the stew. It is more and more unusual for the package meats to have bone included. Red meat is also high in phosphates so it not only does not supply any calcium, but causes calcium to be lost. Americans are aware of the red meat problems and have lowered the level of consumption dramatically in the last four decades.

Smoking is the culprit in losing bone around your teeth. The reason for this loss is that your body tries to neutralize the free

217

radicals in the smoke by using vitamin C. It has been estimated that it takes between 500 and 1000 mg of vitamin C to handle the free radicals in a pack of cigarettes. The daily recommended allowance is less than 100 mg. Once the vitamin C is gone, the body reacts by inflammation. The chronic inflammation weakens the bone. As the bone is weakening, it causes the teeth to loosen. Smoking can lead to a person losing their teeth, even if the teeth are perfect in every other way. That is a high price to pay but it does not seem to deter many people. If they are not deterred by the threat of lung cancer then losing teeth will not do it. If you smoke, you need to add vitamin C to help protect you until you quit.

The gradual loss of bone around the teeth and the chronic swelling (inflammation) of the gums make nice homes for bacteria. The more bone that lost the harder the teeth and gums are to clean. These deep areas are called pockets. The deeper the pockets, the worse the bacteria become. All sorts of nasty little critters can live undisturbed in deep pockets. Even amoebic parasites can be found. Regaining healthy gums and bone is a hard battle to win. Holding your own is the best you can do.

The level of calcium loss to be called osteoporosis is 30 percent, the same amount of loss required for a cavity to show up on an X-ray. Osteoporotic bone is also brittle. Fluoride makes tooth enamel harder but also more brittle. Fluoride makes the skeletal bone brittle, too. That is why areas that are fluoridated show a higher incidence of hip fractures. You may think that a broken bone is not too serious, but statistics show that 20 percent of people who are hospitalized for a broken hip never go home again. For many people it means that their freedom of movement is permanently over, a serious problem. Fluoride is not worth the risk.

On the other side is how to get your bones to be stronger. The recommended level of calcium in the diet by the federal government has been increased several times and is now up to 1500 mg per day. That level is fine except it does not go far enough. Calcium does not exist in a vacuum and requires magnesium and vitamin D to be absorbed and utilized correctly. Products are available on the market with all three components in one tablet.

Vitamin D has been gaining favor as it is now thought that many Americans are deficient. Our bodies make vitamin D when we are exposed to sunlight. Some times of the year we cannot easily get enough sun exposure in the northern part of America. Other people stay inside the year around. The fluorescent lights to which we are exposed in most businesses do not give us the right wavelengths of light to make vitamin D.

You can try to get as much exposure to sunlight as possible up to a half an hour per day. Using full-spectrum fluorescent bulbs can be a big help in your office space. Taking supplemental vitamin D can help. The prescription form of vitamin D cost about $5.00 per hundred in the early 1990's. The price rapidly escalated to $90 per hundred for no obvious reason, since it is inexpensive to make. (Dr. Clark gives the technique in her books.) As a child we were given small capsules of cod liver oil in the winter; that shows the need for vitamin D has been know for at least 50 years.

Calcium also requires stomach acid to put it into an ionic form so it can be better absorbed. Recommending the use of Tums (TM) as a source of calcium forgets that its purpose is to neutralize stomach acid; it also contains aluminum. Check the label. Other calcium tablets are made from animal bones so it has high levels of lead. Not good. Some sources are literally rocks.

And we do not digest rocks. A possible good source is enriched orange juice, except many people are allergic to citrus fruits.

The Dairy Dilemma

Dairy products are always touted as the ultimate source of calcium (by the Dairy Council). The pros and cons of dairy product consumption are a whole book in itself. Many people cannot tolerate milk sugar (lactose) because we lose the ability to make the enzyme lactase as we age. We start losing lactase at the age of two. It is difficult for Afro-Americans to tolerate dairy products, as they are often lactose-intolerant.

Dairy products have so many problems that each person must research it for themselves. Do not be swayed by their clever ads with milk moustaches and "Got milk?" You can bet that many, if not most of the people shown in the ads do not drink milk. Athletes are often told to avoid milk before games or meets as it is a mucous-forming food and may reduce their abilities. Your body produces mucous when trying to prevent something from being absorbed into the body; that should tell you everything you need to know.

Children with milk allergies and allergy caused dental problems are the ones dentists see most commonly. Young kids, age's three to eight, often are seen with dark blue bags under their eyes. Clogged sinuses are also seen routinely. To find out if it is milk requires taking the child off of all dairy products for two weeks to see if the symptoms go away. All dairy products include ice cream and cheese. Butter is OK.

What happens to children with milk allergies is that their sinuses get clogged. They begin to breathe through their mouths.

220

The sucking of air through the mouth tends to alter the face by making it long and narrow. The palates may become highly arched. The dental arches (where the teeth are) become narrow and crowded. To correct some of these conditions, braces are needed, one of the reasons so many of our children are in braces. Braces are not common in countries that eat a more primitive (natural) diet.

It is now the position of pediatricians that children under one year should not drink cows' milk. No other mammal (we are mammals) drinks milk (nurses) after they double their birth weight. Americans are now being nursed at a much higher rate than when nursing was actively discouraged after WWII; that is also the era when the use of orthodontics grew to become common.

Bottom line is that it is better for babies to be nursed and should be nursed as long as possible. Most children will wean themselves. After weaning, milk should be used sparingly. If you are buying gallons of milk, you should be looking for the problems it causes. If you or your children crave milk, then you can be certain there is an allergy going on. If you are Afro-American, avoid milk or take lactase enzymes to help you body cope.

People with calcium absorption problems may have large amounts of calculus (tartar) build up on their teeth. Many patients will have visible amounts of calculus within a week of a dental cleaning. Much of this calcium comes from their skeletons. Their biological calcium mechanisms are out of balance. There are so many systems that it is difficult to figure which system is not working, or maybe all of them. Trying to supply your body with the essential vitamins and minerals gives your body the best chance of righting itself.

In many cases, it would be best to see a nutritionally centered physician who can do blood work analysis. Many dentists want to do analysis and some have tried, but the dental boards have been quite stern in stopping such services. The dentists are thought to be practicing medicine and are told to stop or lose their license. Many other kinds of alternative practitioners are helping people find the true cause of their health problems.

The Process of Tooth Decay

Enamel, the outside of the tooth, is made of dense calcium crystals and a bit of organic matter. Beneath the enamel, making up most of the tooth, is the dentin, which is less dense, with more organic matter, and is full of tubules (little tubes). Under a microscope, the dentin looks as if it was made of pipes cemented together (See Fig. 1.2, page 13).

Decay occurs when the enamel and the dentin of the tooth break down. This breakdown happens by the action of bacteria and their waste products on the molecules of calcium in the crystals. Once the calcium molecules are lost, the crystal disintegrates. As millions of the crystals break down, the area turns from being harder than bone to the consistency of peanut butter.

Other Calcium Loss

When calcium is lost from the bone, we call it osteoporosis. When calcium is lost from the teeth it is called decay and could be called "dentinoporosis," taking a loss of 30 percent of the calcium to cause either osteoporosis or decay. The major difference between osteoporosis and tooth decay is that bone can regenerate and teeth cannot. Therefore, the bacteria can continue to take advantage of the initial breach and cause further breakdown of the tooth. Decay will continue until the conditions causing the decay are eliminated or until the tooth becomes abscessed (gangrenous). An abscessed tooth can continue to breakdown but once it has abscessed, it is beyond saving (See Fig. 1.4, on page 15).

The reason teeth decay is that they have lost the ability to protect themselves from attack of the bacteria and their waste products, and this loss of self-protection is caused by diet. The key food that causes this damage is sugar, but you already know that. It is not a lack of brushing, flossing or fluoride that causes decay. The sugar causes internal systemic changes that stop the tooth's natural defenses.

Accepting Decay

Thanks to the profit motive in modern industrialized countries, tooth decay has become a way of life. We are constantly under pressure to choose a diet that promotes decay. However, since we can choose a diet that causes decay, we can also choose one that prevents decay; that is a profound statement. Decay does not sneak up on us; WE INVITE IT IN!

Our decay-causing diet is also the basis for the profession of dentistry. If there had been no decayed teeth, the profession would not have evolved. This underlying fact may mean that dentistry does not have a real interest in the eradication of decay since it would be like "biting the hand that feeds them." There is an old saying, "You dance with the one who brung ya." Thus, dentists are the bastard stepchildren of the sugar industry.

Although the dental profession as a whole has a vested interest in treating the results of decay, instead of fighting the cause, individually, many dentists may have great interest in seeing the end of decay. These dentists are the ones who talk about diet, not crowns; who talk about vitamins, not gum surgery; who talk about prevention rather than treatment. These dentists are motivated to change their patients' attitude toward diet. Unfortunately, no dentist gets paid to prevent decay, only to fix it.

Likewise, food sellers do not make their money telling you what not to buy. The economics are against telling you the truth about healthy diets. Governments, too, will always be more influenced by those that reap profits through concerns about jobs with campaign contributions of "money for influence" deals. That will always be the way of the political world. You are the only one who can look out for you and yours.

Preventing Decay

The emphasis on fluoride use as a way to prevent decay may be an example of the shortsightedness of the government and the dental profession. The majority of dentists believe that supporting fluoridation of the water supplies shows they are interested in preventing decay. While that thought may be noble, the concept is flawed in many ways. First, fluoridated water may not really work as well as you have been told. Second, fluoridation causes toxic side effects to your body and the environment, which is the reason most European countries have abandoned the use of fluoridation of their public water supplies. And third, the approach is based on "having your 'Coke' and drinking it too". The idea that we can abuse ourselves with a poor diet and at the same time protect our teeth with fluoride is wrong. The idea that we can eat foods that are damaging and yet protect certain areas of our bodies, like our teeth, is contradictory to whole body health and will not work because everything we ingest can affect every part of our bodies. Inconvenient as it is for dentists, our mouths are part of the rest of our body.

While decay is a complex problem affected by one or more factors, including the amount of plaque present, the acidity of the saliva and our individual ability to handle the amount of sugar we eat, the most critical factor is the amount of sugar we eat which negatively impacts each of these each factors. By significantly reducing sugar levels in your diet, you eliminate virtually all chances for decay.

Of the 20 or so different kinds of diets in the world, Dr. Weston Price found that only Western diet, which is high in white flour and sugar, is damaging to our teeth and facial development. With these many other diets to choose from, that means we can enjoy many foods without suffering the damage of major dental problems.

Unfortunately for people in other parts of the world, the U.S., instead of learning other people's healthy ways, is corrupting them by exporting the American way of life, including our sugar-based diet. For example, 80 percent of all carbonated beverages are now being sold outside America. (If you reverse that statistic, Americans, who make up only 6 percent of the world's population are drinking 20 percent of the carbonated beverages, which is still three times the world average per person.) In a short time, the teeth of a billion people will be destroyed in the name of corporate profits. No amount of dentistry will be able to help these people. There are not enough dentists in the world to handle even a small percentage of the damage that is occurring.

If the governments of the world wish to protect their people, they need to stop licenses to import or bottle our soft drinks. They should ban our candy as well. They will not take these steps, though, because it is not in their leaders' economic interests, as import license fees and product royalties are lucrative. It is only in the people's interest to ban the sale of these products. If we cannot educate our own people to the dangers, how can we do it in dozens of languages in a hundred countries?

Reversing The Trend

The saving grace in this overall problem is that decay must have continuing supplies of sugar to keep growing. If a person corrected their diet, then any decay would stop growing. Dentists call this "arrested decay." Even decay around old fillings can stop growing if the diet improves.

Teeth can heal themselves, but cannot make themselves whole. Destroyed enamel cannot be regrown. Teeth will still need repair. Dentists will always have work even if there never was another cavity. If we concentrate on the young, cavity-free people, we could have a generation that grows up to be adults without any decay.

It be done, but must be done by example. Adults idolize brand-name soft drinks and candy bars who cannot tell the kids they are bad, just as we cannot tell them to stop smoking when we still smoke. We must decide that short-term profits are not worth long-term health damage. For a start, supermarkets could eliminate the gauntlet of candy through which we push our carts to reach the checkout.

National Sugar Holidays

Another way we can alter sugar habits is to break the connection between sweets and holidays. Halloween is a dietary disaster for our children! Valentine's Day and chocolate, Easter and marshmallow rabbits, Christmas and candy canes are just as bad. Again, thanks to the profit motive and our national character, we do tend to overdo everything. Moderation and common sense need to prevail. Then perhaps, some day, in about 50 years, the need for dentists will be minor. The controversy about filling materials will fade because there will be no fillings. The need for crowns and root-canals will also disappear (except for accidents). The fluoride can be removed from our water and dental home-care products. "Plaque" will be a word found only in old textbooks. Dentures and denture adhesive commercials will slowly disappear from our lives.

The only requirement for all this to happen is that we, as a nation, begin to eat more in harmony with our body's needs. But YOU DO NOT HAVE TO WAIT! You can begin today. For you and your family, a dentist-free future is possible.

Locations of Decay

Decay is a symptom of a problem, and knowing where it occurs, we can better address its cause. While there are large underlying nutrition causes, there are also more local problems, such as people who clean their teeth well except the back corner of the upper second molars; a cavity there can be avoided by slightly improving cleaning habits. But if many teeth are found with decay at a routine check-up, then there may be underlying problems in diet, health or hygiene. To just fix the decay and not find the cause will doom more teeth to the same fate.

Occlusal Surfaces

The most common place for a cavity is on the chewing or "occlusal" surface of the molars. On this surface are natural pits and fissures (grooves) left from the formation of the tooth. If you look at a molar without decay, they may appear as black lines. The black is stain but decay may also be present. There may be decay in these fissures in some people as soon as the tooth comes in (erupts). Most people's teeth take a bit longer to show damage, depending on diet. This type of decay can be delayed or prevented with the use of sealants. In most other countries with a more coarse diet these surfaces are polished smooth by chewing.

Since the enamel is harder and more resistant to decay, the decay in any occlusal cavity can only penetrate into the tooth through these pits and fissures and begin to spread when it reaches the dentin. Decay moves more quickly through dentin than it does through the enamel because of the dentin's open tubules and lesser density. (The more rapid spread of decay in dentin applies to decay in any location, not just occlusal cavities.) Decay is always more extensive than it appears, either visually or in X-rays. Occlusal cavities, especially, may become quite large without a person knowing they are there. Often the first time a person finds the cavity is when the enamel breaks while chewing.

Interproximal Surfaces

The side of a tooth that touches another tooth is called the interproximal. Therefore, an interproximal cavity is one that occurs between the teeth, usually just below where the teeth touch (the contact point). This is the area that can only be cleaned with dental floss. This decay is best detected by taking "bitewing X-rays."

Smooth Surfaces

Smooth-surface cavities occur on the sides of the teeth that face the tongue or the cheeks or lips, usually near the gums, partly on the root. These cavities commonly happen during the mid-teens when soft drinks are more popular than oral hygiene. Many adults have teeth with white lines in these areas where the enamel was attacked but the cavity did not continue and the enamel rehardened after their diets improved. (Remember, decay is reversible when the cause is removed.)

Root Surfaces

Although decay in a tooth usually occurs in the enamel, decay can also occur on the surface of the exposed root. The root is composed mostly of dentin, the same dentin that is under the enamel. In normal decay the enamel breaks down and then the dentin is attacked. Wear and tear occur as we age and the top of the root is exposed. Since the root does not have a hard protective layer like enamel, it can be more vulnerable to damage, including decay. However, exposed root surfaces will not begin to decay simply because they are exposed; if that were the case, no one would have teeth. Root decay, as with any tooth decay, is diet dependent.

Dry Mouth

Root decay happens more in older people not only because they have more root surface exposed and more risk factors, but also because they have had years to damage the dentin from exposure to bacteria and unhealthy foods. In many older people, a significant risk factor for root decay is "dry mouth" or "xerostoma" caused by medications. Over 300 different prescription drugs may cause dry mouth as a side effect. It is not unusual for older people to take 6 to 10 medicines on a daily basis, both over-the-counter and prescription drugs.

Having a dry mouth hurts the teeth in two ways. First, not enough saliva is available to dilute and neutralize the acids produced by bacteria. This is the case where chewing sugarless gum may help. Second, saliva re-calcifies damaged teeth and inhibits bacteria. Without saliva, the teeth have little or no natural protection, and tooth destruction can be quite rapid.

For example, a middle-aged man who was taking a diuretic (water pill) to lower his blood pressure destroyed his beautiful teeth in less than a year by sucking on "lemon drops" which he thought would stimulate more saliva. The sugar in the lemon drops fed the bacteria that produced acids, which quickly destroyed every tooth.

In another case a man who had his lower salivary glands removed because of cancer began drinking a popular soft drink and chewing sugared gum to relieve the dryness in his mouth. In less than six months he had destroyed four teeth and had cavities in five more, leaving only nine teeth out of the sixteen. The solution was stopping the use of sugar to prevent further damage. The best he could hope for was patching the damage where possible and getting by with fewer teeth, because replacing the teeth with dentures is not an effective solution as the dryness makes wearing dentures difficult.

These are examples in which dentists see the patient after the damage is done. When it comes to medications, dentists are powerless to interfere with the physicians who are treating "more important" problems. If a prescription drug is causing the "dry mouth," the prescribing physician may be able to switch a patient to another drug that will be less damaging. A dentist cannot do more than tell the prescribing physician what is happening in the patient's mouth, but dentists do not normally contact a patient's physician about dental problems. Physicians need to watch their patients for oral damage caused by their medications, but rarely do, relying rather on their patients to tell them if they are having problems. If a patient does not complain, the doctor will not know anything is amiss; therefore, it is important for patients to tell their doctor about any and all side effects they are experiencing.

Whatever its cause, root decay is a never-ending problem. A major problem is that root decay is not isolated. When the factors are right for the root dentin to break down, all the exposed dentin of a tooth, or even the whole mouth, can be affected. The root decay may be deeper in one area of the tooth, but there may be no dentin that is not damaged.

Repairing Root Decay

A dentist trying to repair the root with a filling means there is nowhere to place the edge of the filling where it will be in good healthy dentin. With the edge of the filling against weakened dentin, the decay process continues, leading to an early breakdown between the dentin and the filling. The filling does not last very long before it must be replaced with a larger one. However, placing a larger filling becomes a problem, since the dentin of the root is not very thick. There is not much depth before the nerve canal is reached or is there much room to place a filling before the surface curves around to the side. Thus, placing ever-larger fillings becomes impossible, as there is no more room in the dentin to hold the filling. Crowns do not work any better than fillings because they break down around the edges, too.

Another problem in treating root decay is that bonded fillings do not bond as strongly to dentin as they do to enamel. Bonding uses the calcium crystal structure that make up the tooth. Dentin, being less dense than enamel, has fewer calcium crystals on which to bond. As "dentinoporosis" (decay) occurs, the calcium crystals to use as bonding sites become fewer and fewer.

There are no easy answers once root decay occurs. The use of the prescription drug Peridex may help by controlling bacteria. Keeping the plaque off the root will keep acid levels lower. The amount of bacteria can also be reduced by using baking soda and hydrogen peroxide, separately, to clean the teeth. Topical fluorides and fluoride rinses may slow the process but will not stop it. The toxicity of the fluorides on bones must be considered, since current research shows fluorides actually weaken bones, increasing hip fractures.

Proper Nutrition Is Critical

However, there are nutritional answers or at least help. It is critical to cut down on sugar use. The first thing that has to go is soft drinks, both regular and diet. Eliminate all obvious sources of sugar, like in coffee and tea. Any sugar consumption should be with meals followed by brushing. Try to eliminate hidden sugars by carefully reading food labels. Avoid snacking. Chewing sugarless gum can help curb the urge to snack and may even help by stimulating the salivary glands. Do not use sugarless candies.

Most dentists are not trained in dental school to give nutritional advice. You can tell the dentists who do not know much about nutrition because they will only advise you to "eat a balanced diet." If you ask more specific questions, most dentists will not have answers. Some dentists, though, have learned about nutrition since they graduated, and will give you specific recommendations.

Mainly, you will have to rely on yourself to find information about good nutrition for oral health. Use the library to find books with current information, go to the bookstore, or borrow books from friends. The best advice is to eat whole foods, as raw as possible, like the proverbial "Apple a day keeps the doctor away."

Two Puzzling Phenomena

We are all told that if we do not brush and floss, we will get tooth decay. One puzzling phenomenon that occurs is when a cavity is found on the side of a tooth that touches another tooth, the decay usually in just one of the teeth. Logically, if decay is caused by food left between the teeth being turned to acid by bacteria, the decay should affect both teeth, since both teeth are exposed to exactly the same food. Both teeth are brushed the same, flossed the same, and have been equally exposed to any fluoride products used or water drunk. If brushing, flossing, and using fluoride had any effect, then both teeth would be affected equally. Since only one tooth seems to be affected, there has to be another critical factor. That factor is the tooth's internal resistance to decay; one tooth has it, the other does not. The obvious questions are, "Why is one tooth stronger?" and "How can we make all teeth as strong?" Yet, because these questions are never asked, they never get answered. We are told to brush better and eat less sugar. It seems like we have "missed the boat" by blaming plaque for causing cavities.

The second phenomenon is when another cavity forms, it is commonly on the same tooth on the opposite side of the mouth. Even more curious, this is not just any cavity, but one in the exact same place and usually the same size. That cavity cannot have anything to do with plaque or brushing, flossing, and using fluoride, but must to be due to something affecting the ability of the matching tooth to resist breaking down.

This phenomenon can only be explained if there is a connection between the two teeth and something else that is inhibiting these teeth's ability to resist, indicating that connections to other parts of the body may exist that influence the health of the teeth. If so this concept shows that the teeth are an integral part of the body. If the teeth can be hurt by a problem elsewhere in the body then the other parts of the body can be influenced by what is happening to the tooth. It is a two-way street.

This is an important concept that ties the practices of dentistry and medicine intimately together. Dentists ignoring the effects of their treatments and materials must learn to see the effects of their treatments. And physicians must take into account what dental treatments their patients have had and how these treatments can affect or cause medical problems.

Mercury fillings, root-canals, or whatever else is done to a tooth will cause trouble in other parts of the body. This far-reaching concept should lead to decades of research. Some of this research has been going on in other countries, particularly by the late Dr. Voll of Germany. It is important to acknowledge these phenomena here in the U.S. and take an active role in further research.

What Dentistry Needs

The majority of mercury-free dentists are only opposed to using mercury, ignoring or minimizing problems with other metals and techniques, such as nickel and root-canals. By substituting composites and gold for mercury, it is the same game, different materials. What dentistry really needs is a complete, objective review of all procedures and materials, in which each procedure and material is examined against an ideal standard. Only those procedures and materials that are the most biocompatible and have the fewest side effects should be allowed. If nothing close to the ideal can be found, no treatment should be done. Saying, "It's the best we've got." is not good enough. The standards for acceptable procedures and materials must be raised.

Furthermore, for every procedure and material that meets the new standards, an "Informed Consent" form should be created. When a dentist proposes using a material, the appropriate Informed Consent would then be given to the patient so he would know exactly what could happen. Patients need to know the pros and cons of their treatments. Optional procedures, such as crowns and cosmetic dentistry, should be clearly distinguished from true needs.

This review of procedures and materials will not be popular in the dental profession, for it will reveal the many "skeletons" hidden in dentistry's closet. Dentists should not fear it, though, because it will raise the standards of the profession, making them less dependent on selling high-cost procedures, like crowns, to make a living. Most dentists will welcome that!

Universal Precautions

To prevent the spread of disease among health care providers and their patients, The Centers for Disease Control, a federal government agency, established the concept of "universal precautions." This concept states that all patients should be treated as if they had a communicable disease, such as HIV/AIDS or hepatitis. Since it is impossible to know for sure if someone is a carrier, the best way for a health care provider to protect himself and his patients is to assume that everyone is infectious.

In the dental office some of the precautions are very visible. Dentists use new gloves for every patient, wear masks and eye protection. Other precautions are less obvious but just as important. Equipment, for example, must meet certain standards. Everything possible should be disposable. Every instrument disposable must be sterilized by one of several standard methods every time it is used. Certain equipment that cannot be sterilized must be thoroughly disinfected. Every surface possible should be covered with a disposable wrap, and exposed surfaces that cannot be covered must be disinfected. Clothing worn by dentists and staff members must meet certain standards and be cleaned in certain ways. Wastes must be treated and then disposed of in specific ways.

Most of these universal precautions are common sense and reasonable. Although it took a few years to get used to all the changes, most dentists follow the guidelines closely. After all, their lives are at stake, too! Perhaps the biggest adjustment for dentists was getting used to working in gloves. Working dentists at one time proudly called themselves "wet-fingered dentists." Now, they call themselves "wet-gloved dentists." Dentists are now comfortable wearing gloves and would never work without them, even if they could. Many dentists wonder how they ever survived the exposure risks they took when doing surgery without gloves. Looking back, it seems very primitive and naive to think that they could routinely work in blood and get by with just washing their hands.

Hidden Expense

The use of universal precautions has not been without significant costs in both time and money. The federal government estimates it costs less than $1,000 per office per year but the new equipment alone costs thousands of dollars, even $10,000 per office. The disposable equipment alone comes to several dollars per patient visit. But the staff time maybe the biggest expense. It is estimated by the ADA that full compliance with universal precautions have added over $20,000 per year per office which totals nationally over 20 BILLION dollars in new health care costs. Of course, these costs are passed along to the consumers, just as the cost of every other government-mandated regulation must be. Nevertheless, at a total cost per patient visit of $10, it is a bargain if it protects you from any kind of cross-contamination.

As a patient, you have a right to expect that the universal precautions are routinely followed and to ask questions to be sure. No one is sure if all of these regulations protects patients. But if they have saved even one person from getting HIV, they may be still worth the trouble for the peace of mind.

Cycles of the Immune System

Whenever there is any trauma to the body, be it a major injury or having a few mercury fillings replaced, the individual may experience certain after-effects. Post-traumatic reactions that occur because of dental treatment have been described by Dr. Huggins. These reactions tend to occur on the seventh, fourteenth and twenty-first days after the trauma or dental treatment. While not everyone notices symptoms, about half the patients do report reactions similar to the beginnings of the flu, which are actually the immune system getting ready to protect you. Patients report feeling weak, "off," depressed, and tired. The following morning they feel fine. Symptoms usually worsen with each of the seven-day cycles, then stop. This cycle repeats for each appointment. Therefore, you should not have appointments on the same day of the week within a month of each other.

If you try to have your work done on the same day for four weeks in a row, the effects of the cycles will be added on top of each other, making you feel ill and weakening your immune system. Thus, you should avoid repeating days, even if you must delay treatment. It is also important to write down the dates of the cycles for the three weeks following each date of treatment. If you have four appointments you would have 12 days to watch (3 days for each appointment, therefore 3 X 4).

It is also best not to push treatment during any given appointment. It seems to work well to limit dental work on any day to two hours, usually enough time to do one-fourth of the work for the average patient. For a patient needing eight or fewer fillings, it might be enough time to do half of the work.

Systemic Infections Caused by Dentists

Lip service is paid by dentists to the fact they may cause systemic (body-wide) infections from what they do, but more and more physicians know this. In a book on risks to your longevity an M.D. states that periodontal disease can shorten your life by 3.5 years. While it acknowledges that dental infections can shorten your life, the numbers may be off, as it is quite possible that a dental infection may not just shorten your life but end it.

Preventing oral bacteria from getting into the blood is a common warning that has been given to dentists for decades. It should not be news that flooding the blood with bacteria in even a healthy patient is a bad idea. Such a flooding comes during a dental cleaning when the gums are swollen. Patients with excessive bleeding should be on preventive antibiotics, as well as flushing with antimicrobial rinses before and during treatment. A massive influx of bacteria of a hundred different species can overwhelm the body's white blood cells.

If this is so dangerous than why do we not hear about people getting sick? Normally, the bacteria in the blood do not cause trouble immediately, but several days later, which means most people do not connect the two things. People do not think that dental work can be that traumatic. Famous people who have had troubles illustrate the point. The famous country singer, Waylon Jennings, had to cancel some concert dates due to a dental infection. Wilt Chamberlain died a week after he had two infected teeth removed. His health failed after the extractions. He may have died on the seventh day (See Immune Cycles). There is little doubt that dentistry pushed his body over the edge. Elvis Presley had his teeth cleaned the day he died. Makes you wonder, doesn't it?

Veterinarians have brochures in their offices detailing what can happen to your pet if they have infected mouths spreading bacteria into the blood. The booklets tell of liver and kidney damage. Dentists have brochures telling patients about infected gums as well, but these talk only about loss of bone and gums tissue, not life-threatening consequences.

It does not even have to be a full-blown gum infection to be dangerous. An infected wisdom tooth can damage the heart. Any abscessed tooth can overwhelm the immune system and make a person listless even in the absence of pain. The infection may even be worse if there is no pain. Pain means the body is trying to contain the infection and cause it to come to a head and drain. An infection without pain means the body is not isolating the infection so the bacteria are escaping continuously into the body, creating an ongoing burden for the immune system, including the lymph glands and liver.

If you are otherwise healthy, you may be able to function and not even know the infection is going on. If something else requires your immune system to protect you, then there might not be enough strength left to do both jobs and your health declines rapidly. The body fights to eliminate the bacteria and their toxins;

if it cannot remove them, it isolates them as best as possible to protect itself.

These bacterial toxins will build up first in tissues that are regenerating the fastest. The female reproductive system is very vulnerable. Chronic sinus problems are as common as root-canals. Many patients claim immediate sinus relief after years of suffering once the infected tooth is removed.

The links to oral infections are obvious if someone looks for them. If the dentists are totally focused on fixing teeth and gums, they can be blind to what lies beyond. If they do not see the connection for you, then you must see it for yourself. People ignore the dangers coming from their mouths at the peril of their lives.

Dental Cleanings

It has been a mainstay of dental practices that people should see their dentist twice a year for a checkup and cleaning. This practice started early in the century and was attacked by many dentists of the day as a way to get patients into dental offices when they did not need treatment. It was the custom of the early dentists to have open waiting rooms, where patients with problems would come and wait their turn. Many dentists of the day thought that doing a dental checkup was akin to stealing patients' money for doing nothing.

A strong case can be made that prevention is the best dentistry. Regular cleanings may help prevent gum disease but it can also cause damage to the teeth. It can be argued that routine check ups have been changed from a help to a patient to a source of profitable elective procedures. It is touted by practice management seminars as a way to motivate patients to accept the "best dentistry has to offer." What that really means is selling crowns to patients.

Another profitable procedure management consultants tell dentists to promote is "root planning." Root planning is deep cleaning at a much higher price tag and insurance coverage. Whether root planning is a real benefit to the patient can be argued, but the financial value to a dental practice can be substantial. There is a real possibility that permanent damage can be done the roots and gum tissue, the opposite of the purported purpose of the treatment.

It is not unusual for patients to complain that having their teeth cleaned is an ordeal that creates painful teeth and bleeding gums for days and weeks after; this should not be the case. If a twice yearly cleaning is an ordeal then you should not have them. You must decide what is right for you. You can spend more time in your daily cleaning techniques to reduce the need for professional cleanings. If there is too much bleeding during brushing or professional cleaning, then a serious gum (periodontal) problem may be present. Aggressive cleaning by a professional at this time may be dangerous, even fatal. Special care must be taken.

Dr. Hal Huggins does not believe routine cleanings are necessary. These cleanings may not be needed for everyone but that depends on the person. Some patients who do an excellent job cleaning their teeth still like two cleanings a year. Some people build up calculus (tartar) quickly, while others never have any. Other people need to get cleanings done twice a year to maximize their insurance benefits. Two key points: The diet is the real threat to teeth and you are in charge of your own mouth.

One common thing is people's confusion about the term "plaque." This confusion seems impossible when this term is in a million toothpaste ads every year, but I doubt if 10 percent could correctly define it. Most people think plaque is the hard deposit that the dentists or hygienists clean from their teeth. Those deposits are calculus or tartar. Plaque is the white gooey stuff that coats our teeth, the film that we feel in the morning when we reach for the toothbrush, the film we can scrap off with our fingernail. Try it now!

Plaque is inevitable and no matter what we do, will always be there and actually, is supposed to be there. Plaque only becomes a problem when we change it with our Western diet, which changes it from a protector of the teeth to a disease-causing condition when our sugar-laden foods stimulate it's overgrowth. It is the Western diet that has transformed our need for food into a disease-causing crisis, but that is another book in itself.

It is not important for a dentist to remove the plaque because it can never be completely removed and will quickly reform. Usually a day is sufficient, that leaves 5 months and 29 days until the next dental cleaning. Therefore, it is critical that we do our best to keep the plaque to a minimum with complete daily cleanings.

Patients often say with pride, "I brush twice a day." Be still my beating heart--two times a day! That is better than one patient who thought he brushed at least once a week. Not one of my patients ever said that they brush after every meal even though this is the standard advice. In a perfect world, one well-done cleaning at bedtime would be fine. Since such is rarely the case, brushing after every meal is not a bad idea.

Saying, "brushing" is not quite right. Brushing is the least critical part of cleanings because most of the real problems occur between the teeth where the brush does not reach. Does the word "flossing" ring a bell? Most patients dislike flossing and many cannot do it for a variety of reasons. It is almost universally true that people who clean their teeth well, including flossing, have the healthiest mouths.

To tell if your mouth is healthy, check a couple of obvious signs. The color of the gums must be a light pink. There should be no bleeding when flossing and brushing. The tongue should be pink, and not have a yellowish coating. You may find stains on the teeth, particularly when you use various herbs and tea. Stain may be unattractive but is not dangerous.

It is important that the teeth be checked. The more fillings you have the more important routine checkups are. The most dangerous problems are cracked fillings which leak, allowing decay to start under the fillings and packing food between two fillings allowing decay to begin on the root. Either problem can destroy a tooth before the person is aware of it. X-rays may be necessary to see this damage. It is common for patients who have had their fillings changed to skip the next several routine checkups. Please do not.

X-Rays

Two major schools of thought exist on what are the basic X-rays needed for an examination. The technique taught in dental schools is the full-mouth series, 20 small X-rays covering varying views of all the teeth. While this type of X-ray supplies good information on the teeth it misses many other structures. The second technique involves taking two bitewing X-rays, looking for decay between the back teeth and a panoramic X-ray that is 5 inches by 12 inches, showing all the structures from one ear to the other and from the eye sockets to the Adam's apple.

The panoramic X-ray gives a view of the sinuses, wisdom tooth areas, below the roots, the edge of the lower jawbone, temporo-mandibular joints (TMJ), and the ability to compare right and left sides for differences. It is important to have a panoramic X-ray; there is no substitute.

Patients have learned that getting X-rays is not a healthy idea but they have over learned. Dental X-rays are a minor assault on the body that has been lessened over the years by reducing the amount of X-rays actually needed to expose the film, the use of lead protection devices and keeping the taking of X-rays to the minimum needed to get the information necessary to do the examination.

It is quite possible that a person getting a good amount of vitamin C (over 1000mg) will not be affected at all. Vitamin C protects us from free radicals that X-rays create. It is appropriate to tell the dentist you are concerned about getting X-rays and you want them only when they are directly requested by the dentist. If the dentist believes they are needed and the patient refuses to get them, the dentist should not continue the examination. Dentist are liable for correctly diagnosing problems and without current X-rays they are blind to many problems. A dentist may feel that the patient is questioning their competence, which may damage the rapport needed for a good doctor-patient relationship.

It is almost unheard of for a patient to refuse an X-ray requested by a physician even when those X-rays are much more dangerous that dental ones. Patients must believe that their doctors have taken this possible danger into consideration when requesting X-rays; if they have not, then maybe the patient needs to find another professional to do their work. Refusing to have an X-ray that the dentist has personally requested either directly or through his assistants must be a red flag to the dentist. He should stop treatment until the matter is resolved. If upon further discussion the patient still refuses and the dentist still believes he needs the X-ray, then the patient should seek treatment elsewhere.

It is important that a reasonable basis for taking X-rays be part of a health-based practice. A panoramic X-ray should be done only every five years unless there is a specific need. Bitewings are routinely done on a yearly basis for people with many fillings. In people with few fillings and excellent oral health, having bitewings taken every three years is not unreasonable. Any longer than three years is not advisable. If you have many fillings, it may be unwise to not to have yearly bitewings done. Only in extreme cases would bitewings be needed more often than yearly. A missed new cavity may destroy a tooth before it is found in any other way.

A new type of X-ray equipment is coming onto the market, called digital X-ray, which uses computer sensors instead of film and need as little as a tenth of the present amount of X-rays to get an image. These X-rays are close to the quality of film-based X-rays. The systems are many times more expensive but will come down in price. Within a decade they will probably become the standard, as young dentists equipping their new offices will start with digital X-ray machines.

Many patients have to take their X-rays for many reasons. There is much confusion on this issue. The law dictates that patients have a right to their X-rays but not the originals. If the dentist has not done any treatment, then there is no reason he cannot give the patient the originals. If any work has been done, then the dentist needs to maintain the X-rays in his records, but must be able to supply the patient with copies of the X-rays. The dentist is allowed to charge for this service. The copy is never as good as the original and a new dentist cannot use it to make a diagnosis or should you want him to do so.

New Technologies /Lasers

Lasers are high-intensity beams of energy. That can be used in dentistry to vaporize tissue. Properly adjusted and used, these beams can vaporize at low temperatures and one cell layer at a time. With such ability lasers can coagulate tissue so there is no bleeding when gum tissue is removed. In many incidences, laser beams can even be used without anesthetic. Lasers are also being touted as a way to sterilize root-canals. (Remember, there is no such thing as a sterile dead tooth.) There are several types of lasers, each with specific applications. To fully utilize lasers in the dental office, more than one type would be necessary, further increasing the costs.

Lasers may have many beneficial uses and in a perfect world every dentist would have one and be an expert in its use. As with other technology, the application is far different from the promise. Few dentists are expert in its uses and it will stay that way for quite a while if not decades. There are limitations to its uses and these limitations guarantee it will remain for the next generation a very-high priced toy, not a routinely used technology.

Lasers cannot be used for many procedures. The beam cannot remove metal fillings or crowns. The beam may form volatile toxic compounds when it hits tooth structures, contaminated with previous filling materials (metals). Lasers cost quite a bit, as much as equipping a whole room with the regular dental equipment such as a chair, light, cabinetry, normal hand instruments, handpieces (drills), and an X-ray machine. Unless they can be used often enough to justify their costs the dentist will lose money. After doctors buy an expensive piece of equipment, they tend to find ways to justify its use and the fees necessary to cover costs and expected profits.

Until more affordable lasers are available that are less technique-sensitive (i.e., hard to use) and reliable, few dental offices will use them. If your dentist has a laser, do not be surprised if he does not find you need some type of laser treatment. Use your common sense about it. Ask about the alternatives and costs of the laser treatments before you agree. While he might be "the dentist," it is still your money and you get to choose what is done to your body.

Air Abrasion

Air abrasion, a technique unsuccessfully introduced in the 1950's, has made comeback with updated technology. Air abrasion uses a high-pressure stream of air with particles of aluminum oxide to cut the tooth structure and seems to work best on small new cavities, so is commonly used by children's dentists. Commonly used without numbing, it is a fast technique and when coupled with flow able composites, quite profitable.

Most dentists have resisted adding air abrasion to their practices in spite of these obvious advantages. Many of the units are quite expensive and is also technique-sensitive. The right tip, the right air pressure, and the right angle all have to be used or the tooth may be damaged. Some dentists do not like blasting aluminum oxide particles into the air they breathe. Special suction equipment must be used to keep the splatter to a minimum.

Most fillings are replacement fillings. While air abrasion works quite nicely on composite fillings, it does not work on mercury fillings, which are the majority of fillings needing replacing. Air abrasion has the unusual property of cutting hard tissues faster than softer ones. Composite fillings are harder than the tooth, so it cuts it first. Decay is soft, so it cuts the tooth around the decay, undermining it. If the decay is close to the nerve, an exposure of the nerve can easily occur. Most dentists will see this as another excuse for doing a root-canal, when the decay goes all the way down to the nerve. If you think root-canals are a bad procedure, then an exposure is the last thing you want to happen. Be cautious when its use is suggested.

1-800-Dentist

You have seen the 1-800-DENTIST commercials. They are well-produced and it would seem any reasonable person wanting to find a new dentist would be tempted to call, so they could "match you with a qualified dentist near your home." It seems generous of them to do this. You might wonder who sponsors these commercials and why.

These are reasonable questions. Here are the answers. It is a company who wants to make money. They make money not from people who call but from dentists who pay them a substantial monthly fee for them to tell callers their name and address. The system is done by Zip Codes. The first dentist who signs up gets the area. Callers are matched with the dentist who pays them, actually is not much of a matching process.

It seems that this service would be a natural for a mercury-free dentist so when a patient looking for such services called, they could be matched to my office. When we inquired, they said it did not work that way. If we paid their fee, we would have all the referrals that came from people in my Zip Code, not just people looking for the services our office provides.

If you want to find a dentist who does the type of dentistry discussed in this book, you need not bother to call 1-800-DENTIST. If you do not have a dentist you know, then you will need to get out the Yellow Pages in your city or area and start looking. Some dentists advertise "white fillings" or "cosmetic dentistry." You should call dental offices and ask questions. You may need to interview dentists to find an office that suits you. The internet may also be a help. Just use some common sense.

10

WHAT TO DO? WHAT MATERIALS TO USE?

Compatibility Tests For Dental Materials

Compatibility tests are done to check the reaction of your blood to various single components of dental materials. The concept is that if your blood cells react to the material, it is probably a bad one for you. If the cells react a little, the material may be tolerable. If the cells do not react at all, it is assumed to be safe for you to use.

A large number of dental materials are made of many components. The compatibility tests examine the components rather than the material itself because this is simpler to do than to check thousands of different materials that have similar components. It is reasoned that if you react to a component, then you will react to the complete material. Thus, any material that has the tested component in it is given the same rating. For instance, if you react to barium silicate, every material that has barium silicate as a component is marked as reactive. The reasoning is that by using only materials to which you do not react, that is, materials with which you are compatible, you will protect your immune system.

Accuracy of the Tests

Compatibility tests are recommended by many anti-mercury dentists and physicians. This method of testing seems reasonable and may have value, to the point of being essential for some sensitive patients. But before the concept is accepted as valid, key questions need to be asked: 1) Are the tests reliable? And 2) Are the tests consistent? At this time the answers to these questions are a qualified "maybe."

It may not be accurate to assume that if you react to a component of a certain material that you will react to the complete material because when it is within the whole material the component may become inert or trapped so it will not affect the person. This reaction is a major drawback to these tests. Another big problem is that your test results may change after the mercury fillings have been removed. If your body's immune system is weakened by dental materials already in your mouth, you may test sensitive to a material that by itself would not cause a reaction. But this reactive material may be the best material available for use, if the immune system is not already weakened. If the test was repeated six months after you have had your mercury fillings changed, the material previously listed as "not acceptable" may then be "acceptable."

The only way to find out for certain what materials may be the best is to remove all the metals and replace them with temporary fillings. After six months without mercury a compatibility test would be done. You may have more confidence in those results. The problem with this method is that patients do not want to go to the trouble of having the work done twice. Who could blame them?

Further Considerations

Another problem is when if you have a compatibility test done and it recommends several composite materials as "non-reactive," that is, safe to use, your dentist may not have any experience with those materials. These materials may even be composite materials that the dentist believes are less desirable, because of their poor physical properties or handling characteristics, and he may not wish to use them. It is up to the patient whether to use the recommended materials in spite of the dentist's objections. If the patient insists, the material may have to be specially ordered, which will probably cost a bit extra or the dentist may refuse to do the work if he has to use an inferior material.

Even then the test results may not be 100 percent reliable because the results are only what was found with that particular blood sample and that a blood sample one day later may give different results. At about $350, the full test is not inexpensive. You may wish to contact the lab for the latest information on the tests and an explanation of the reliability of the test before you make up your mind.

Reducing Exposure To Materials

It is better if you can keep the total number of materials used to an absolute minimum. If you use only one composite material, you reduce your risks of reaction. The tests are more useful to dentists who do metal crowns and root-canals, because they are using many more materials. If you are not having those "not recommended" procedures done, then most of the test information would be useless, anyway.

253

Dental materials can also be tested for compatibility in ways that exceed the scope of this book. Many dentists may use these other methods instead of a blood compatibility test, but they may or may not be more reliable, and they may be more reliable if done by one dentist over another. As you can tell from the lack of a firm answer to the questions about reliability and consistency, there is no black and white choice. It is a matter of using a combination of techniques to find a compatible material.

A disturbing finding is that there are contaminants in all dental materials. It is too expensive to have any product 100 percent pure, so each metal used contains tiny amounts of other metals. Mercury may have thallium and/or uranium in it; both can be debilitating. Whenever any metal is used, you have to assume that there will be other metals tagging along. No one knows what a given material might have; it may change from batch to batch. The only way to protect yourself completely is to have perfect teeth with no fillings. Second, would be to remove all teeth that have had a filling and the gums surrounding them. The next way would be to eliminate any form of metal in the materials chosen. Any other choices are more risky and no one can tell exactly what danger you may face. In American crown metals, it is not necessary to report any metallic element that is in a concentration less than 2 percent. It has also been reported that all gold used contains some nickel.

Recommendation: If you are sick to very sick, a compatibility test may be worth taking because very sick people do not have any reserves, any room for error. Using a material that is reactive may reduce or eliminate your recovery. If you are not sick, only concerned, the test should be done only if you would feel more secure if you take every precaution. In the latter case, the odds are in your favor that after six months, you will be doing fine with or without the test.

For most patients, the risk is small that a particular composite will be a long-term problem. The biggest problem is usually the mercury fillings. Once these fillings are gone your body begins to detoxify itself. Although it can take years to get all the mercury out of your tissues, the total mercury burden will decrease daily. As it decreases, the body begins to right itself.

Meridians

Meridians are based on the Chinese Qi (Chi) or energy flow channels. Along these energy channels are specific spots (gates) that can be used to stimulate or block the energy flow. These channels and spots are the basis for the 5000-year-old practice of acupuncture. They are routinely used by many alternative practioners that use EAV (Electro Acupuncture – Voll) machines. Chiropractors and kinesiologists use these channels to diagnose and treat patients.

Dental meridians are the same meridians as acupuncture and acupressure meridians. Hostility and derision were shown to those who first brought the concept of acupuncture to America. After decades acupuncture has become partially accepted by American mainstream medicine. Physicians may not understand how it works but they can see that it does have value. The use of it in dental situations will become accepted eventually.

The work on dental meridians was done in Germany by Dr. Voll. While it is not an accepted practice to try to diagnose using Dr. Voll's chart, it is a tool to consider as to how a dental infection may be affecting someone's total health.

People wonder why there are meridians, what purpose can they have, and how they came to be. If one meridian can be explained, then it is reasonable to accept that the others probably exist and their origins will be discovered eventually. It is commonly accepted that there is a connection between dental infections and problems at remote locations. A dental infection, even a cleaning where there is infection, can send bacteria into the blood stream. It can even be fatal to people who have damage on their hearts valves. The reverse can also be found in the medical/dental literature. A heart attack can cause jaw pain. With this two-way street it is not surprising to see that the wisdom teeth are on the heart meridian.

The meridian that is most easily understood is the one dealing with the eight front teeth: four on the top and four on the bottom. This meridian chart lists the urogenital system (that means from the kidneys down) and the lower bowel. Dr. Hulda Clark told me once that when she was a little girl, her mother told her that if she had to use the rest room she could stimulate the urge to release urine by sucking on her upper front teeth. You may want to try this but it might be best to do this when already in a rest room.

When you think about how this meridian might have originated, think about how a baby nurses; it sucks. The sucking stimulates the bowels to move, keeping the baby regular. This function still works in many adults in that they need to use the rest room while they eat or shortly after. Observe this when you are in a restaurant. Sucking also works with animals. Our dogs need to go out right after they are fed.

One way to use the dental meridians is to check the critical teeth: wisdom teeth or extraction sites, root-canals and abscesses. You can look for areas that seem to be weak in your own case and see if there are any infections, root-canals, or cavitations on these meridians. Another area that needs research is the effect of the electrical charges from metal fillings and crowns and how they affect the meridians.

There are some meridians that are of particular concern. The teeth on the breast meridians should be at the top of that list. These teeth are the upper first and second molars and the lower first and second bicuspids. These are common teeth to have root-canals. The chronic infections in such teeth will drain into the lymph system and weaken or infect the breast. The other meridians that seem to be commonly found to negatively effect the body are the four meridians that go through the wisdom teeth, which affect the heart.

Dental Meridian Chart

Most of the recent books on alternative dentistry contain a dental meridian chart. These charts are hard to read as they have to be shrunk to make them fit the page size, making them more difficult to see and understand. Patients have been given charts four times larger in our office for years. Problem teeth have been circled and the meaning of the chart explained. It does not seem that patients can grasp what the chart shows. A glazed look is often detected. It is confusing enough for people to learn the common names for the teeth but for them to transfer it to a chart and make sense of it probably is asking too much. To try to make it more clear, only the major effects of groups of teeth are listed below. Since the chart cannot be used for diagnosis, this will give you an idea of what problems can occur elsewhere in the body from dental sources.

The worse problems come from abscesses, traditionally a swollen tooth but also from teeth treated with root-canals and unhealed areas in the bone called cavitations. There can be large effects from electrical charges created by all the metals that can stimulate or block a meridian. It is all very complex, so complex that it can only give us indications, not certainties. The organs affected will be on the same side as the tooth, e.g., a root-canaled lower right bicuspid would affect the right breast. Below is a sampling of some of the most important effects from dental meridians. The key area of effect is capitalized.

Wisdom teeth:	HEART, lower back, small intestine, energy
Molars (upper):	BREAST on same side, sinus, stomach
Molars (lower):	LARGE INTESTINES, neck, lungs
Bicuspids (upper):	BREASTS, large intestine, lungs, neck
Bicuspids (lower):	BREASTS, stomach and esophagus
Cuspids (all):	EYES, gall bladder and liver
Front teeth (all):	KIDNEYS on down, lower bowel, sinuses, adrenal glands

Not every person has a major problem such as cancer. It is common for patients to tell us that after a particular appointment, some change occurred. More than one patient has told us that a pain they have had for years in their big toe went away. Another said that his "anal itching" stopped. Who would go to a dentist because they had anal itching? Another said her panic attacks stopped. Who would go to their dentist to treat panic attacks? These examples show the profound influences of dental materials.

Enamel Rating

The outer layer of the tooth, the enamel, is the key to keeping a healthy tooth. Ideally, the enamel will remain intact for the life of the person. In our country the enamel is under constant attack from our sugar-based diet. As it is damaged, the dental profession repairs it with a variety of materials and techniques. Each technique requires shaping or removing various amounts of the enamel.

Each technique described in the book will be given an "Enamel Rating" on a scale from one hundred to zero, depending on the percentage of healthy enamel left. One hundred would mean all the natural enamel is left undamaged and zero would mean no enamel is left. For example, a sealant does not require removal of enamel and gets an enamel rating of 100 and a crown would require that most, if not all, of the enamel be removed, so it would get an Enamel Rating of 5 or less.

This Enamel Rating will give you a tool to better judge the impact of different treatment options a dentist may recommend. You should protect your tooth enamel from unnecessary damage, both from eating and cleaning habits, as well as dental treatments. The better you care for your tooth enamel and the less dentists do to it, the better off you will be. Remember, before having any dental procedure done that requires removal of any enamel, think long and hard. Remember, NO DENTAL TREATMENT IS PERMANENT BUT DAMAGE DONE TO TOOTH STRUCTURE IS FOREVER.

Sealants

Sealants are a plastic coating used to seal the pits and fissures on the chewing surface of teeth and on the sides of the molars. Sealants are the same material as the plastic used as in composite fillings. This material penetrates the deep pits and grooves, physically sealing them from bacteria and food. If bacteria and sugar cannot easily get in, then the tooth has a better chance to mature and harden.

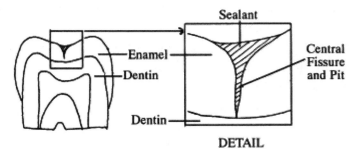

Sealants

Figure 10.1

Sealants seem to be effective in preventing decay and are recommended routinely for the first and second molars. Sealants are most effective when placed when the molars first come in, which is around age six for the first molars and age 11 for the second molars. Sealants can be placed can be done on other teeth, including the baby molars and the permanent bicuspids if there is a high risk of decay. If the child eats poorly, work hard on improving the diet, as it will have the more profound impact on the child's total health. In the meantime, use sealants wherever reasonable to protect the teeth. For an enamel rating: 100, no change in enamel is necessary.

Rubber Dams

The rubber dam is a thin sheet of latex or vinyl that can be put around the teeth being worked on to isolate them from the rest of the mouth, so that the materials removed do not get in the saliva and the saliva does not contaminate the filling while it is being done.

Although the procedure for using rubber dams is taught at every dental school, and has been for decades, but not all dentists use them. There are many important reasons to use the rubber dam, but most important is to keep the mercury particles out of patients' mouths. Once the mercury is out, many dentists remove the rubber dam, as it may hold mercury particles near the gums. Some dentists then place a second rubber dam, to help control moisture.

It is occasionally impossible to place a rubber dam as the teeth are so close together that it will not fit. A few people are claustrophobic and cannot stand to have one placed. Even if you think it might bother you, it is worth at least an attempt to place a rubber dam to find out how you react. Most people like to have them used. They are highly recommended.

Potential Problems

One of the main problems with the dams is they become tiresome for the patient during long procedures because their mouth has to remain open at all times. A rubber dam can be taken off and replaced easily. Replacing mercury fillings, for example, may take an hour or two per quadrant and patients really need to stop and rest at half-hour intervals to keep the procedure from being too much of an ordeal.

261

Another reason not to use a rubber dam is that the clamps that hold the rubber dam in place are uncomfortable and stress the teeth on which they fasten. These teeth may ache for days after the procedure. Teeth that have weak bone support need to be avoided as sites for clamping.

Another hazard is that the rubber dam holds mercury particles around the edges of the teeth next to the gums until after the dam is removed. Mercury vapor can even penetrate the dam just as it can the latex glove the dentist wears. Sometimes patients will be sensitive to the latex or the fragrances placed in it to hide its odor.

Since there are pros and cons to the use of the rubber dam, a recommendation that one be used every time is not possible. While in general one should be used, it is not always a good idea or even possible. A diligent dentist can work without a rubber dam. Since each case is different, discuss it with you dentist before work is scheduled.

Anesthetics

The most common anesthetics used in the dental offices are 'shots.' The most common comment dentists hear is, "Nothing personal, Doc, but I hate dentists." Actually, it is the shots they hate. Much is done to make numbing as pain-free as possible. Many new gadgets are being marketed to make it easier. As a patient, you need to accept the fact that in getting dental work done, there will be some discomfort. You need to look past any discomfort to your goal of getting the metal out of your mouth. Anything you can do to make it less stressful to the dentist works in your favor. Keep your nervousness as much under control as you can. The best way to get an injection is to close your eyes, relax, and keep breathing slowly and deeply.

It is important which anesthetics are used. The most common is lidocaine with 3 percent epinephrine. The epinephrine is the medical term for adrenaline. It is the epinephrine that gives some patients a rapid heart rate during or right after they get the injection; this normally passes in a minute or two but it can be very disturbing to many people.

The purpose of the epinephrine is to close down the veins that would move the anesthetics out of the area to be detoxified in the liver. It holds the anesthetic in the area longer so that the numbing is deep and long lasting.

There are some problems with epinephrine. Besides the chance for a rapid heart rate the most common side effect is from the preservative that is used when the epinephrine is added. The preservative is sulfite, a very common allergen; it gives many people headaches which patients blame on the stress of having dental work done.

The other side effect of the restricting the blood flow can be reduced healing after dental surgery. Low blood flow may be a minor problem while having fillings done but during extractions, having good blood flow is critical. Your body needs to bring fresh blood into the area to bring oxygen and white blood cells. The white blood cells are critical in fighting the bacteria that always get into the socket during and after an extraction. (See Extraction.)

Almost every dentist has several anesthetics on hand, one of which should be epinephrine-free. You may request that the dentist use epinephrine-free anesthetics in most every circumstance. If you tell the dentist that you are allergic to anesthetics with epinephrine, they will not use them. The generic names of some of the most common anesthetics used are lidocaine, mepivacaine, and prilocaine. Epinephrine-free forms of are each available. Ask about what anesthetics are available when you first call or at the examination appointment.

It does happen that some patients do not get numb, get numb slowly, or only get half-numb with epinephrine-free anesthetics. There are many secondary techniques to numb, so you do not have to suffer through any pain. If you tend to numb slowly, please tell the dentist at the first examination appointment so extra time can be allowed. Do not accept enduring pain for the sake of the dentist's schedule. Dentistry is hard enough but it is much more stressful for both you and the dentist if you are feeling pain. Even if it only hurts a little bit, the pain can change to unbearable in an instant. Bravery is not necessary. Dentists are usually under time pressure so if a patient takes too long to get numb, it may destroy the schedule. It is in your best interest to minimize causing the dentist any undue stress. Dentists do better work when they have enough time available. If they are behind and have two patients waiting, they cannot do as good a job as if there was plenty of time available. It is also better if the dentist can concentrate on doing your work rather than going from patient to patient. If you find things are getting out of hand, you can ask to be rescheduled.

Some dentists delegate the actually filling to expanded duty dental assistants. A dental assistant may be able to do a good job, maybe even a great job but the odds are against it. Doing a good composite filling is difficult. The ADA states that the technique sensitivity (hard to do) of a composite filling is one of the two reasons dentists do not use them. If it is hard for a dentist who is supposedly highly trained, then how could it be easy for a dental assistant? It is difficult to find a dentist who can place a good composite. Finding a competent dental assistant would be even more difficult.

Bases

The new composites are designed to be used directly in contact with the dentin and are designed to bond to the dentin. It is this bonding directly to the dentin where many problems occur. The worse is postoperative sensitivity to hot, cold and pressure. Most of this type of sensitivity can be eliminated with the use of a base under the filling. The manufacturers of new composite materials promote how little post-op sensitivity occurs with their product, indicating sensitivity was at least a problem in their earlier products.

Another benefit is that when the filling is to be replaced, it is easier to see the difference between the base and the composite. If the filling is bonded directly to the dentin, it is difficult to tell one from another. For accuracy, it must be mentioned that many bases contain zinc, but this seems to be compatible with most every patient. It has also been noted that finding decay under an old base is unusual, so they may have some anti-caries property.

If your dentist does not use bases, that is okay. With new materials and the rapid change in bonders, the use of bases is not essential, but may be worth having done. Such bases take much extra time so paying an additional fee is to be expected. It is worth it.

One class of bases is called glass ionomers, heavily promoted but containing properties not recommended at this time. Avoid their use.

Zinc oxide and eugenol bases have been recommended by Dr. Hulda Clark as fillings. These fillings are considered temporary fillings; they may last only six months to a year but do a good job as a temporary. The bases have two major drawbacks; one is that they are not strong and can be broken out within a year and second, eugenol is not compatible with composite fillings. It might not be possible to bond a composite filling into a tooth later on, if there is any eugenol contamination. It is also not considered a good dental practice to leave patients with a mouth full of temporary fillings, even if it is their express wish. Such is the effect of having a society driven by lawsuits.

Calcium Hydroxide Bases

A calcium hydroxide base is a compound placed under fillings because it is thought to stimulate the tooth's cells to the wall of the dentin tubules, thereby helping the tooth protect itself. Dentists are taught to place them under all fillings as a matter of routine, believing them to be beneficial; this is not the case.

Calcium hydroxide bases should not be used routinely because one of two things generally happens: The compound can either be absorbed into the tooth or it becomes mushy (like cottage cheese) by absorbing moisture. Either way, the filling is undermined and becomes weaker. Furthermore, composite fillings gain strength by bonding onto the enamel and dentin. Covering the dentin with the base reduces the amount of surface available to be bonded by more than half.

The use of calcium hydroxide bases is an example of "cookbook dentistry." Since dentists have always put calcium hydroxide bases under their mercury fillings, when they switch to composites, they tend to keep doing everything the same, only changing the filling material. Switching to composites is not easy, because composite fillings require their own technique from beginning to end.

Generally, a calcium hydroxide base should not be used routinely and never under a composite unless there is a direct exposure to the nerve. While this may seem too technical for patients to worry about, it is included because many patients are seen who have had their mercury fillings replaced with composites which fail because the dentist put calcium hydroxide bases under them. By avoiding the mistake in the first place, patients may save considerable trouble and later expense.

Pins and Alternatives

Pins are small threaded posts used to strengthen large fillings, which dentists call "pin-retained fillings." For example, when a cusp breaks off and not enough tooth structure remains to hold a filling, a pin is one way to add the necessary retention. The pins most often used are really self-tapping screws. A small hole, slightly smaller than the pin to be used, is drilled into the dentin of the tooth. The pin is then screwed into the hole, cutting threads in the dentin as it goes. Pins come in many sizes from so small that they are hard to pick up, to very large ones used inside root-canals. Pins are made from several different metals. The least expensive and weakest are a gold-colored brass, the strongest stainless steel. The newest, most expensive, and most biocompatible metal pins are made from titanium.

267

Pin Problems

Using pins sounds like a great technique, but it can cause many problems. Using traditional dentistry's cookbook approach, any problems caused by pins are fixable with other, more elaborate (and more expensive) treatments. Before you have any pins placed, you need to "hear the rest of the story."

One of the biggest problems with pins is that they exert tremendous pressure on the tooth when screwed (tapped) in. The mechanical driver turns the pin until it locks up and twists off at a weak point on the top. The torque (pressure) created can put a hairline crack in the dentin, which is difficult to locate but can ultimately lead to the loss of the tooth. The crack can go from the pin to the outside of the tooth, which can let anything found in the mouth leak into the tooth, corroding the pin. Or the crack can go from the pin to the inside of the tooth where the nerve is, beginning a breakdown that ends with the tooth dying. Pain is also possible from a hairline crack. In most cases, an internal crack leads to the death of the tooth, and unfortunately, hairline cracks are common, occurring on the average of once for every three regular-sized pins. If the tooth does die, the dentist may believe it was because the tooth was already in weak condition before any treatment. True, the teeth most likely to crack are the brittle ones, which are brittle because they are already dying or dead. For this very reason, the use of pins is ill-advised.

What else can happen when a pin is used? The dentist can miss-drill the hole. The hole must be placed with great care between the outside and the inside of the tooth.

Because this area is narrow, it is difficult to fit the hole in the middle. If the angle is off or the access is difficult or the hand and eye of the dentist are less than perfect, the hole can be drilled either right into the "nerve" or right into the outside. Either place is bad, but if the hole goes into the center of the tooth, the nerve, it means either a root-canal or an extraction. Of course, the dentist will want to do a root-canal and then a crown for "protection and strength." A ten-dollar pin just turned into a thousand dollars worth of treatment. Good for the dentist, but not so good for the patient.

Very Small Space Available

To give you an idea of the maximum size of the space a dentist has to work with when drilling the pin hole, look at the crossbar of this "t", which is about 2 millimeters wide or a twelfth of an inch, a bit wider than the width of the tooth where the dentist must place the hole for the pin. On one side is the outside and on the other is the "nerve." There is little room for error. If all goes well, and it usually does, the dentist drills the hole halfway from either side. Remember that this drilling is being done inside someone's mouth, and if it is on an upper tooth, it is being done upside down in a mirror. You can imagine how easy it is for something bad to happen.

If a dentist inadvertently drills into the nerve, you would think he would not charge for any additional treatment needed. Think again. A dentist would never use pins if he had to take responsibility for any damage they caused. Although your attitude may be that if the dentist causes a problem he should fix it, it does not happen that way in either medicine or dentistry. It is not a perfect world; treatments on teeth do not always go as well as hoped even for the most skilled dentist. And it is sometimes difficult to tell if a treatment goes bad because of circumstances, lack of ability, or just an unusually shaped tooth. This is why dentists need to discuss the consequences, both good and bad, that are possible, as a result of using pins. "Informed Consent" forms should be used.

Can Pins Be Replaced?

"What happens next?" That is the question this book is trying to get people to ask before any treatments are done. This question needs to be asked for every treatment, every time. The importance of the question is seen when it comes time to replace a filling containing a pin. It is common to see corrosion around the pin caused by mouth fluids leaking under the filling or though a crack. In most cases the pin cannot be reused, so the dentist will just cut it off leaving the embedded end. In metal-free dentistry no pins are used and the whole pin must be removed by drilling the embedded end out; this is very intricate work.

It is difficult to redo a pin-retained filling. The more pins in the tooth, the more difficult it is, because it is difficult to remove a filling and not have the pins come loose or be cut off. Why not put in new pins? It is impossible to keep putting in new pins because there is now less tooth structure to hold them and the best places were used the first time.

For a traditional dentist, once a pin is used, the path to needing a crown is set. He will usually suggest doing a crown because the tooth is so "weak." In fact, many dentists only use the pin-retained filling as a way to build up the tooth to hold a crown. Their recommendation is to go right to the crown "before the tooth breaks down and needs to be extracted." But crowns have problems as outlined in their own chapter. (See "Crowns.")

A pin-retained filling can last 10 years, but there are ways to rebuild any tooth without using pins and have it last just as long. Virtually any tooth can be rebuilt using the bonded composite fillings.

The Proper Bite

The way your teeth come together is called your bite. When you have dental work done, it is common for your bite to be changed but it is important that it returned to its original feel. The most common thing to happen is that the new dental work will be too "high," meaning it is the first place that strikes when you close your mouth. Dentists try to get the bite right by having the patient chew on a piece of marking paper, a type of carbon paper which shows which place hits first. The dentist then adjusts these places, until all the high spots are gone.

Unfortunately, often patients are unable to tell the dentist how it feels because they are too numb. In addition to not being able to fully feet the bite, the muscles may be affected by being numb or just from holding the mouth open. Therefore, it is difficult for patients to get a natural movement after being worked on. If they are not sure if it feels right, it may be best for them to stand up and loosen up tight muscles.

Patients will often try to be helpful and say it is all right when it is still too high. It is very important that both the dentist and patient spend all the time necessary to get the bite returned to a comfortable condition because a bite left too high can cause many problems. The most minor result is that the tooth will become sensitive to cold. But if it is off enough, the constant mis-hitting can cause inflammation inside the tooth which can lead to the tooth dying.

Patients have difficulty communicating how their bite feels. They seem to expect it to feel different, when it should not feel different at all. Besides saying that it feels "high," patients may use terms like "full" or say that they cannot feel their teeth on the opposite side. Sometimes getting it right might be frustrating for both the dentist and the patient, but it is important not to rush the process. A minute or two now may save coming in for another appointment to correct the bite.

Different Materials

The various dental materials react differently if the bite is left high. With mercury fillings, if the high place does not break off, the material will slowly squish away because mercury is a liquid. With composites, which are permanently hard once the light cures them, are so hard that they will not wear quickly enough to prevent a sore tooth. A crown is even harder. In fact, crowns are so hard it is difficult to get the bite accurate, so opposing teeth are routinely damaged.

Because of the potential for damage, it is important for the patient to tell the dentist if their bite feels wrong. Even if it requires a return trip the bite must be corrected. Patients tend to not want to "bother" the dentist and think that if they wait a few weeks, the problem will correct itself. But it is not worth damaging a tooth hoping the problem will go away. A patient should not delay getting a high bite corrected.

Light-Cured Materials

A revolution in dental materials began 20 years ago when light-cured composite materials were first marketed. The material comes from the manufacturer containing a light-activated curing agent. This means that no mixing of separate components is necessary. Instead, once the dentist places the material in the prepared cavity, a bright light is shone on it for about 20 seconds, which activates the curing agent and hardens the material.

Before light-cured materials were developed, chemical curing was used. The hardening process was achieved by mixing a chemical activator into the material, leaving the dentist with only about two to three minutes to place the material in the prepared tooth. If the placing of the material was not finished before it began to set, it would have to be removed and redone. The warmer the material, the faster it sets.

Advantages of Light-Cured Materials

Some important advantages to "light-cured" materials over "chemically-cured" materials are: 1) No mixing is required, so the material is always exactly the same; 2) the material does not set until activated by the light, so the dentist has all the time necessary to get the material exactly where it needs to be; 3) more material can be added to previously hardened material because it chemically bonds to itself; 4) the material is much more color-stable and does not darken with age; 5) it lasts longer; and 6) it can be repaired.

Early Use of Composites

When chemical-cured composites were first available, many dentists tried them in back teeth with poor to disastrous results. For one or even all of the drawbacks these early composite fillings were doomed. Failing quickly, they caused considerable damage, including abscesses. Dentists felt that by using the composites, they were causing more damage than they were solving any problems that the use of mercury fillings might cause. These bad experiences left many dentists opposed to using composites in back teeth.

Dentist were right in their opposition, because chemical-cured filling materials should never be used in back teeth. This early experience may have prevented dentists from trying the light-cured materials when they became available.

Until the mid-1980's most dentists did not have light-curing systems in their offices. While the initial systems were introduced around 1975, they were taken off the market by the FDA because of possible ultraviolet light damage to the eyes of the dental staff. Dentists who had these UV lights had to switch to the new systems, which use a white light. Many dentists, were wary after losing money on the UV lights, decided to wait to see if anything went wrong with the new lights before buying one. In the 20 years since the new light-curing systems have been on the market, they have proven to be the superior to all other filling systems, but there are still dentists who do not own or use light-cured materials. These dentists are in the dental "Dark Ages." If your dentist does not routinely use light-cured materials, get another dentist because he is too far behind to do good work for you.

Composite Materials

Which composite your dentist uses might be very important. Many people seeking mercury are sensitive to other chemicals. Some chemicals may be in one composite and not another. Trying to determine which composite or other dental material might be better for you is the purpose of compatibility testing. If you are sensitive then you might want to give serious consideration to having a test done. (See COMPATIBILITY TESTING.) Of the other methods, such as, kinesiology and EAV or electro-dermal testing, individual dentists may use the most chemically inert filler for composite filling materials is quartz. Most new composites do not use quartz, but various glasses and ceramics that contain heavy metals which are added so the fillings show up on X-rays, making it easier for dentists to tell the difference between the tooth, filling, and possible new decay. The heavy metals added are barium, strontium, and zirconium, the most common being barium. Barium does leach out of the fillings and is associated with breast cancer. Remember, in the mouth, everything leaches.

If you really wish to be metal-free then the composite you use must be metal-free. There are not too many composites without heavy metals because the dentists want them to show up on the X-ray. Dentists are used to seeing the mercury fillings and it is more comfortable for them to see the composites the same way. The goal of the ADA and material manufacturers is to have a composite that handles just like mercury fillings so dentists can switch effortlessly.

The material used in our office currently is one of the original composites named Visiofil by Espy; it does not show up on X-rays and is also the material that shows up on virtually all the compatibility tests as acceptable. The newer composites are being continually altered to make them easier to use and stronger, but that does not make them more biocompatible.

There may be many other composites that contain no metal, but is no such list is available. It may also happen that Visiofil stops being the composite of choice in our office. It may even be removed from the market if the sales are not high enough. The current material used in our office will be placed on our website (**www.dentistry-toothtruth.com**). Please check the site before you encourage a dentist to use any particular material. If the dentist does not use the material listed, he should be able to buy the material you want. Do not be offended if he charges you extra to have a special material just for you.

Sensitivity

It is common patients to experience some postoperative sensitivity to hot, cold and/or pressure. This sensitivity is usually of short duration but sometimes persists. If your sensitivity is from pressure or if the filling "feels high," contact the dentist for an adjustment. A tooth can be damaged from constant biting on a high point and can also make the tooth cold sensitive. Do not wait for it to go away. With mercury fillings a high place might go away as the mercury was smashed down. Composite fillings are too hard to be smashed. It is a case of better safe than sorry.

It is possible that a tooth may die after being refilled; this rarely occurs if all the normal safeguards are used. A dying tooth will have a dull ache, often constant. Aspirin or ibuprofen usually stops this pain for a few hours, but need to be used continually or the pain returns. These drugs reduce inflammation which causes the aching. The longer the toothaches, the greater the chance the tooth will not survive. Most dentists will recommend a root-canal; while this will stop most aching, it leads to many other problems. (See ROOT-CANALS.)

Acid-Etch Bonding

To bond is to attach two things together. The perfect way to accomplish bonding is to do it chemically. When a layer of light-cured composite filling is correctly added to another piece of light-cured composite filling, they are chemically bonded and become one piece. However, no filling material has yet been created that can chemically bond to tooth structure, so the process of composite filling is best described as consisting of two types of bonds: the physical bond between the tooth and the filling material and the chemical bond between two layers of filling material. Through the use of both physical and chemical bonds, the composite materials can be firmly attached to the tooth.

To bond a composite filling to the tooth, the surface of the enamel is prepared by etching it with an acid solvent, called the "acid-etch" technique. After etching, a bonding agent is applied that flows into the microscopic roughness of the enamel created by the acid. When cured, this creates a physical bond. The composite filling material can then chemically bond to this layer. It is this first layer that forms the critical seal of all composite fillings.

The acid-etch bonding technique has been available as long as composite fillings materials but was not commonly used, as it requires several extra steps which take time. Time is the enemy of dentists when they are in a hurry. To do composite fillings properly, every step must be done and done correctly. Skipping steps to save time means the fillings will not last. Dentists who use composites successfully must be very meticulous and cannot be ruled by the clock.

By 1980 the new composite materials, coupled with enamel bonding using the acid-etch technique, made it possible to place composite fillings in high-stress areas, such as the back teeth. As the composites materials improved over the last decade, it became possible to restore any tooth using these techniques. The importance of good technique in using these materials cannot be underestimated. Poor technique may be partly responsible for some dentists' reluctance to give up their use of mercury filling material and switch to composites.

Gold

A great many anti-mercury dentists, as well as pro-mercury dentists, believe that gold restorations, such as crowns, inlays, and onlays are the best replacement for fillings. They believe gold restorations are worth the extra trouble and cost because of their strength and longevity which may make them the least expensive treatments over a person's lifetime. The dentists who are skilled in using gold can make it seem like using gold is the proper solution, but patients need to consider all the facts before taking this approach.

The use of gold in dentistry predates the use of mercury by thousands of years, as gold dental work has been found in ancient Egypt. Mercury was not used until the early 1800's. Mercury fillings materials became popular originally because it was much less costly than gold dental work, which is still true today. Although many patients will "go for the gold" in their dental treatment, their numbers will still be small compared to the total patient population. Even if gold were affordable to 10 or even 20 percent of patients, it would still not be the answer to the mercury problem.

Costs of Using Gold

To give you some idea of the high cost of gold dental work, compare it to composite fillings. The extra doctor time and lab costs incurred during the making of the gold restorations easily triple the cost of composite fillings. People who have to pay $2000 to change from mercury fillings to composites will have to pay $6000 or more to replace them with gold.

In an article in Dental Products Report, June 1994, it is estimated that gold restorations cost four to five times more than fillings but last only twice to four times as long. In properly selected patients, the cost of the gold over the length of time it is in use is the same as for fillings. If this is true, then it seems the major disadvantage is the up-front cost, which is quite significant to most people. But there are other considerations beyond costs.

Problems With Using Gold

Gold is not free of problems. Besides being considered unattractive by most people, it is still a metal. Metals in the mouth generate electric (galvanic) currents, which also give an underlying metallic taste to your mouth and may cause many problems of which we are only beginning to be aware. In addition, any gold restoration requires more of the tooth structure to be removed than a comparable composite. Furthermore, gold is an allergen to many people. And while it lasts longer in the studies, it is possible

279

that this is because people who have gold dental work done are more motivated to keep their mouths clean. Most importantly, any time a tooth is crowned, that tooth stands a chance of dying. If a tooth is killed by crowning, it is not being saved, but condemned.

Other Considerations

If you are considering having gold work done, it would be prudent to have a compatibility test. (See "Compatibility Tests") This test will help you choose the most compatible gold alloy. No gold restoration is 100 percent gold; other metals are always included. Although some gold dental materials have a high gold content, most are 10 karat (40 percent). Others contain metals that are dangerous, such as nickel. Remember, the higher the gold content, the higher the cost.

If you decide you want gold work, you must be aware of its interaction with any other metal in your mouth. It is best that all the gold work be done with the same gold alloy to reduce interaction. To protect the new gold work, do not have any of the new gold dental work placed in your mouth if you have any mercury fillings left. Mercury is electrically attracted to gold and will instantly begin to contaminate it. Therefore, it is critically important to have all the mercury removed from all your teeth before the new work is cemented, including remnants of old fillings that may be left under the new restorations. Removing all the mercury first need not involve any additional steps, appointments, or costs. Unfortunately, remnants of old mercury fillings are routinely found under gold work, even work done by "mercury-free" dentists. You must be specific in stating that you do not want any mercury left in your teeth.

Double Check

As an additional safeguard ask your dentist to take new bitewing X-rays after all the mercury has been removed but before the gold is in. It will be apparent on the X-rays if any mercury has been missed, even a tiny amount; if it has, the dentist can easily remove it just before cementing the gold work. Be sure to ask for X-rays to be taken prior to cementing the gold work because once the gold is cemented, any mercury left could not be seen on an X-ray.

Composite Resins

For the majority of patients who cannot afford gold or do not want gold because of its negative characteristics, a less expensive replacement is needed. Such a replacement technique must be one that is already routinely done by most dentists. At this time only one category of material even comes close to fulfilling these criteria and that is, composite resins. In any type of restoration where gold can be used, composite can be used at less cost and hazard to the patient.

The resistance to the use of composites seems out of place. The composite material is really a great material just as it is: Allows dentists to take their time to do a good restoration; can last for years and years; generates no galvanic currents; is closer to the cost of mercury fillings than any other material; is flexible in its uses; can be used for changing the color and shape of teeth; is very natural looking; has been in use for over 20 years, and new, improved composite materials reach the market almost every year.

Inlays and Onlays

Inlays and onlays are fillings made outside of the mouth, then cemented or bonded to the tooth. An inlay is placed inside the tooth, like a filling, whereas an onlay is an inlay that also covers all or part of the chewing surface, and therefore is "on" the tooth. The reason onlays cover the top of the tooth is to protect the edge of the enamel from fracture. Inlays and onlays were made of gold until recently, when composite and porcelain materials began being used.

The difference between these two treatments and fillings is in how the dentist prepares the tooth to hold the various restorations. Inlays and onlays must be made in a dental lab before being placed in the prepared tooth; therefore, the sides of the cavity must slope into the tooth. Although this procedure does require more of the tooth to be removed, because of the additional strength of the materials, it is considered an even trade.

Inlays and onlays may be excellent ways to repair teeth, depending on the skill of the dentist and the lab technician who makes them. The technique used is the same whether the material used is gold, porcelain, or composite. The dentist prepares the tooth during the first appointment, making an impression of the teeth to send to the dental lab. A temporary inlay is then made and placed. At the second appointment, the temporary is removed. The inlay, which has been made at the dental lab, is tried in the tooth. If it fits, it is cemented or bonded.

The material chosen is just as important as for any other dental treatment, perhaps even more so because it may last longer and cost more. Compatibility should be the top concern. Gold is the traditional choice; it can be fit perfectly and last a long time if done properly. A porcelain inlay can be a problem because this material is very brittle and chips easily. Porcelain is difficult to work with and may wear down the opposing tooth, whether it is enamel or another type of restoration. A porcelain inlay is best avoided.

The newest material used for inlays and onlays is laboratory-processed composite. Sometimes these are called "porcelain" because they are white, but are not to be confused with real porcelain. Being processed in the dental lab makes it more difficult than a composite filling. Inlays and onlays have many good qualities: All shrinkage is done outside the mouth so the fit well; do not wear down the opposing tooth; are very nice looking and are difficult to distinguish from a natural tooth; and if damaged or chipped, can be repaired with the regular composite filling material. The disadvantages with composite inlays is that they take two appointments and are about three times as expensive as a regular composite filling. But since composite inlays may be the best restorative material available today, they maybe worth the extra time and expense.

Enamel Rating: 50 to 20 for inlays and 40 to 10 for onlays. Both are below a composite filling because of the needs of the technique in shaping the tooth. The additional strength of lab-made restorations may make up for the removal of more of the enamel.

Improving Appearances

Many people, if not most, are not happy with the appearance of their teeth. Even people with beautiful teeth, in perfect position, with no decay, no gum disease, and good color are not always happy. Many may want their teeth to be even "whiter" or straighter. On the other hand, many people who have truly ugly teeth are happy with them because they are healthy. Most dentists would agree that the patients whose teeth need the most improvement in appearance are often the ones least likely to want it.

Many ways can be used to improve the appearance of teeth. Your first consideration should be to decide what you really want and why. Your dentist can help you decide which, if any, of the four main techniques are right for you. Before any of these techniques are discussed, remember that these are elective treatments. Patients can get along without doing anything. Patients always have the right to choose to "do nothing."

Bleaching

If your teeth are straight but not as white as you would like, bleaching is an option. But before you consider the different methods, you need to know why your teeth are not as white as you might like. Do they need a professional cleaning? Do you have habits that contribute to stained teeth, like tea-drinking or smoking? Were they were darkened by the use of tetracycline when you were a child? Is there fluoride damage (fluorosis)?

If you determine that your teeth cannot be whitened by a professional cleaning or changing your habits, then you need to decide which of the three main bleaching techniques you want to use. The easiest and least expensive is the over-the-counter home bleaching kit, which ranges in cost from $10 to $50. The next technique is a dentist-supplied bleaching system. (It is called a "system" rather than a "kit" because it is more expensive.) These systems require the dentist to make a custom-fitted covering for your teeth which holds the bleaching solution against the teeth. Other than that, these systems are similar to the inexpensive, over-the-counter "kits," but will give better results

The third technique for bleaching teeth is done only for serious discoloration. With this method, the dentist or hygienist uses very strong peroxide with a heat lamp. This treatment takes many long, tedious visits. Although it is said that this technique does not hurt the teeth or cause nerve damage, there are no guarantees. Since this is a serious technique that should be used only in the worst cases, you should be cautious. One hazard is that peroxide can release metals from fillings, so this technique should never be used on teeth with metal fillings. A new version without the need for heat has been recently introduced; perhaps this will make the technique safer.

Most patients like whiter teeth, but you can whiten them too much. No matter how white they become, the whiteness will fade over several years and rebleaching may be necessary. No long term studies have been made about the safety of bleaching. Photomicrographs show tiny holes in the enamel. The studies also show that all the bleaching materials do reach the pulp chamber, so they do directly affect the nerve. Short-term studies reveal enough warning signs showing that it is best to be cautious.

Recontouring

Many front teeth are not attractive because of their shape and position. It is often easy to get a significant improvement in appearance by simply recontouring the teeth. A good example is when a front tooth is too long. In just minutes a dentist can shorten a tooth and dramatically improve the appearance. Often lower front teeth are "ragged" looking, overlap and differ in height. By cutting down the highest teeth and shaping the ends correctly, the dentist can make the teeth took straighter. Another common complaint is pointed "eye" teeth. People do not like these teeth to look like "fangs." In a minute these teeth can be rounded without causing them any damage or loss of function (except during full moons!).

Essentially, recontouring reshapes the enamel of the teeth, removing some of its thickness without damaging the tooth. The procedure is minor and numbing is not required because the enamel is usually thick enough to be shaped without causing sensitivity during or after the procedure. Recontouring does not increase chances for decay.

Since recontouring is usually a short procedure, many dentists charge only a small fee for it or include it with the fee they charge for another procedure, such as bonding. If you are interested in this procedure, ask your dentist about the amount of change possible. You can have some recontouring done and live with it a while, then later have more done until you get the look you want.

Enamel Rating: 95 to 98 as only minimal amounts of enamel are removed.

Bonding

"Bonding" is the term used when a layer of composite filling material is added in varying thickness on the front of a tooth to change its shape and color. The material is bonded on to the enamel and sometimes the dentin of the tooth, but no change in the structure of the tooth is usually necessary. Because bonding does not alter the tooth, the bonding material can be removed without harming it. This reversibility is an important advantage to this technique. It is rare for a dental treatment not to damage a tooth.

The technique of bonding originated as a way to fix broken and chipped front teeth. As dentists began to experiment, they found that feathering the edge of the filling past the edge of the cavity gave a better-looking finish. Eventually, they found that covering the entire front of the tooth gave then the ability to change the shape and color of the whole tooth. Often the repaired tooth looked better than the tooth next to it. The patient then would want the other teeth to look as good as the repaired tooth.

Thus, the original term "bonding" has grown to mean the cosmetic improvement of a tooth or teeth. When a patient asks for "bonding," he wants his front teeth covered with composite filling material to improve the looks.

Bonding is simpler to explain than to do. After the enamel surface is prepared by etching, a bonder is applied and hardened by light curing. The composite plastic is then placed on top of the bonder, shaped, then hardened by light curing. More layers are added until the tooth is built up more than is needed. Then comes the hard part--sculpting a new tooth out of the built-up composite, which takes time, patience, and skill.

During the treatment the dentist should do only two teeth, then let the patient look at them to make sure the results match his expectations. The dentist can then change the shape or color to match the patient's expectations. It is important that the dentist's ability match the patient's expectations, or no one will be happy! Sometimes, bonded, teeth end up looking like "Chiclets," those very white square chewing gum candies. This result is not a failure of the technique or material but a lack of skill on the part of the dentist. Bonding, when well done, looks natural.

"Before" and "After" Photos

Most dentists skilled in bonding can show you "before" and "after" photos of their work. You should look at these photos to get an idea of their skill level. If they only show you a glossy book of other dentists' work or how you would look on an imaging computer, you will not know what they can do. Real photographs of their work are best. They may also give you the names of other patients who are willing to serve as referrals.

After the bonding the initial reaction by the patient is that his teeth "feel funny" because they are thicker. (However, they should not look thick!) It takes only a few days to adjust to the difference. It is not uncommon for women to cry for joy when they see the results. Bonding can be a life-transforming procedure; some patients undergo personality changes because they feel more attractive when they smile.

Cost of Bonding

Although the bonding of six front teeth generally takes about two to three hours, costs around $200 per tooth, and is a bit tedious for the patient, particularly if he must wear a rubber dam for two hours, many patients find the procedure well worth the time and cost. The composite filling material can hide defects in color, shape, and position, it is also repairable, if a corner should chip, so it should last for at least 10 years.

Selling Bonding

When bonding first became popular in the 1980's, dentists attended seminars telling them how they could get rich making patients' smiles prettier. Bonding was the "hot" seminar topic. Dentists were told that people would pay more for cosmetic treatment than for routine fillings, being reminded that plastic surgeons make more money than general surgeons because people are willing to pay more for what they "want," rather than for what they "need."

Two problems disproved this theory. First, there were not enough vain people to make cosmetic dentists out of every dentist who was interested. Second, many dentists could not do a good enough job of bonding to be comfortable with the technique. However, the attempt to sell pretty teeth to patients has not stopped. The current "hot" product is a video-imaging computer. Used to make dentists better at "selling" pretty teeth, like computer plastic surgeons use to sell nose jobs. These machines sell for $5,000 to $15,000, and all dental magazines feature many expensive, full-page ads for them and as of 2000, approximately 40 percent of dental offices have added one of these imaging computers; eventually, most offices will have them.

Although these video-imaging computers are marketed as a way to help the dentist sell more "high-quality" dentistry, patients should read that to mean "high-priced" dentistry. Dentists may say that money is not their motive, but the advertisers are quick to point out how many more crowns the average dentist can do, once he has bought their video machines; that is how the machines can "pay for themselves."

Enamel Rating: 95 to 100 because with bonding, very little change in the enamel must be done.

Veneering

Veneering in furniture is covering unattractive wood with a thin layer (veneer) of fancy wood. The process is similar for veneering teeth. Like "fake fingernails" for teeth, a veneer is a thin, porcelain shell made to cover the front of the tooth. An excellent result can be obtained depending on the skill of two people, the dentist and the lab technician. However, before you decide to have any of your teeth veneered, you should be aware of some of the potential problems with this technique, the most noteworthy being its irreversibility.

As with bonding, you should ask to see "before" and "after" pictures of the dentist's own work. You may even want to talk to a patient who has had the procedure done, asking for their opinion and whether they would do it again. Remember, the dentist will only give you the names of his most satisfied patients.

While it is true that many Hollywood "stars" have their teeth veneered (they tend to make their teeth too white), they are doing so because it is required for their close-ups. This need for the illusion of perfection does not apply to most of us. Many people later regret things they did for vanity.

Veneering Techniques

The veneering technique requires that some enamel be removed from the teeth. An impression is then made and sent to the lab technician (who is, hopefully, a highly skilled artisan). At the second appointment the veneers are tried on the teeth. If the dentist is satisfied, he shows them to the patient for final approval. If the patient does not like them, this is the last chance to speak up! If the patient approves of their appearance, the dentist bonds them to the teeth, one at a time. The bonding of veneers is a bit tricky. If one is bonded in the wrong position, it will have to be remade to correct the problem. The teeth should look the same after bonding as they did during the trial approval.

Many other problems are possible with veneers. First, the tooth enamel has to be cut down between 0.5-1.0 millimeters, which is half its thickness. Sometimes, the enamel is ground off clear through to the dentin. It is this removal of some of the enamel which makes the technique irreversible. Also, the teeth are usually shortened so the veneer can go over the end of the tooth.

Second, if a veneer ever chips, it is difficult to repair and if it comes off, it will have to be remade. If the front teeth have many fillings to begin with, veneers should not be used. If new decay develops between the teeth or an old filling under the veneer needs replacing, it is difficult to do without damaging the veneer.

Third, veneers are twice as expensive ($400-800 per tooth) as regular bonding. Two appointments are necessary if everything goes perfectly, more if a problem arises. A major reason for the high cost is that the dentist must pay a substantial fee to the dental lab to have the veneer made.

Finally, there is a toxicity problem which may exist because porcelain is made from aluminum, along with additional metals used as the coloring agents. A compatibility test is warranted to find the least-reactive material.

Although some veneers are now being made from composites, if any enamel must be removed, then they present many of the same drawbacks as porcelain veneers. These problems with veneering may far outweigh any advantages for the patient.

Therefore, before an irreversible procedure like a veneer is done, the patient must think about what might happen if, or more certainly, when the veneer fails. Can the procedure be repeated? Would the next procedure have to be a crown? Would doing the procedure increase the risk of the tooth dying or being lost? With veneers, it is possible to remove them and use bonding to rebuild the tooth, but unlike bonding, it is never possible to go back to your original teeth.

It is recommended that people avoid the technique, if at all possible. Again, if your dentist swears that the technique is perfectly safe, ask him to put it in writing. You will probably meet with resistance, since dentists do not like to put anything in writing, having been carefully taught and constantly reminded never to guarantee their work. Even if they do stand behind their work, they are extremely reluctant to put it in writing.

Enamel Rating: 80 to 60 because 20 to 40 percent of the enamel of the tooth must be removed.

Crowning To Approve Appearances

Before veneers, it was common practice in Hollywood for each new "star" to be given the Hollywood makeover, including getting their teeth "capped" (crowned). But Hollywood makeovers are not recommended for the rest of us.

If your dentist tells you that the only or best way to improve the appearance of your teeth is not with bonding or veneers, but by crowning them, get a second opinion. Improving appearance should never be used as a reason to crown teeth, because crowning a tooth is too damaging to them.

Possible Effect of Crowning

In a typical case history of a crowning a patient in her early thirties complains about the large, unattractive fillings in her front teeth. The dentist suggests that she would be better off with crowns on her four front teeth, telling her that crowns would be "stronger and last longer" than the fillings. She trusts his judgment, plus she has dental insurance that will cover half of the cost. So the four teeth are cut down for crowns, the crowns are made, and placed and look great. The patient is happier; the dentist is richer.

However, nine years later, a large abscess forms on the roof of her mouth. The dentist finds that the two crowned teeth on the right are infected. After a round of antibiotics to reduce the swelling, root-canals are done on the two teeth by drilling through the backs of the two crowns. Unfortunately, the swelling returns because the infection is still in the bone. The patient is sent to an oral surgeon, who performs an apicoectomy, opening the gums above the roots and removing some of the bone so he can see the root tips. He then scrapes out the infected tissue, cuts the root tips off and seals the new root end (usually with a mercury filling). The opening is sewn closed. Although the pain and swelling are reduced, the patient says they never go away completely.

After another year the patients notices the two teeth are moving outward and up, which makes them look shorter, plus creates a space between the front teeth. The root-canaled teeth are still tender. She now hates all the crowned teeth because of the trouble she has had with them, so she asks the dentist to pull all her teeth and make her an upper denture. Fortunately, the situation is not that bad; the only weak teeth are the two with the root-canals. She agrees to have only the two teeth with root-canals removed. But before the teeth can be removed, one of

293

them breaks off at the gum line. The dentist puts it back together with a new bonding cement, hoping it will hold until the partial can be made to replace it. She spends the next six weeks being very careful not to break off the tooth. Finally, 12 years after the crowns were first placed, the patient has two of the teeth removed and a removable partial placed.

The question raised by this typical scenario is: How well served was this patient by having her teeth crowned? Did they last longer than a good bonded filling and were they as cost-efficient? No, they did not last longer and they cost many times more than bonding. Obviously, crowns can routinely cause more problems than they solve, and hundreds of patients may be having similar crowns made to improve their appearance the very day you read this. However, since crowning teeth can lead to the death of teeth which can lead to root-canal therapy and extraction, which can lead to partial dentures or bridges, maybe even implants, it seems too severe a treatment to crown teeth simply to improve appearances.

Recommendation: The first criterion that you should use in choosing a procedure to improve the appearance of your teeth is one which does the least damage to the tooth for the greatest improvement. In most instances, bonding will be the best choice because it needs no changes in the tooth, thereby preserving the most enamel. While veneering can give great results, it does require removal of enamel and is a difficult technique to do well. Crowns should be avoided.

Since bonding is reversible, you can decide to do something different later on, e.g., veneers. But once you have veneers done, it is almost impossible to go back because the removal of the enamel is permanent. Choosing bonding may be the most practical way to keep your options open for future work when new techniques are developed. Since the average dentist may have trouble doing either of these procedures well, be careful who you choose to do your work. It is a good idea to talk to other patients before you commit to any procedure.

11

CROWNING TEETH

A Dentist's Idea of a Perfect Tooth

A dentist will say that a perfect tooth is a whole tooth, with no fillings or gum problems and in its proper position. But this idea of a perfect tooth seems to change once a cavity appears. The mechanical rebuilding of damaged teeth is how dentists earn their living. The bigger the cavity or fillings get, the less the dentist thinks about the natural tooth structure and the more he thinks of artificial replacements.

Most dentists would say that a crown makes the tooth stronger. It does not! While the crown itself may be strong, it takes its strength at the expense of the tooth. The tooth becomes an illusion of an ideal tooth, one created by the dentist. How could it strengthen a tooth to remove all its remaining enamel?

This dental concept of a strong crown protecting the damaged tooth leads to further problems. Degraded by the removal of its enamel the tooth loses its ability to cleanse itself because the natural fluids flow that through the tooth, from the pulp chamber (which most people call the "nerve") to the outside, are blocked by the crown. (See "Dr. Steinman.") While it may seem impossible for fluids to flow through enamel because of its density and hardness, the flow is always present and critical to the tooth's health. The blockage of these fluids may be one reason for some teeth dying after being crowned. Blockage is also a reason crowns come off and need re-cementing. The dental solution to crowns coming off is to use cements that are more resistant to any liquid.

Damage During Crowning

The more likely reason for tooth death after being cut down for a crown is overheating. The tooth is shaped with an ultra-high-speed drill. Just one millisecond of high temperature created by the drill can damage or kill thousands of cells on the inside of the tooth. This drill can also develop a relatively high suction that can literally pull cells from inside the tooth out through the dentinal tubules. So many cells may be killed that they cannot be replaced. The damaged area inside the tooth becomes gangrenous.

As the infection develops, more and more cells die. In several months to a year later, the tooth abscesses, but most dentists think this is only a coincidence or due to the initial weakness of the tooth. They do not realize that the damage could be caused by the very treatment they used to "help" the tooth. Unfortunately for patients, dentists, in their zeal to make a "perfect" replacement tooth, may kill the real one. Since it is not commonly accepted by dentists that the crowning procedure itself is damaging to the tooth, they do not feel responsible for its death. Dentists believe a dead tooth is not a problem and that a root-canal will make the tooth almost as good as new.

The tooth has now gone from a living tooth with a large filling to an infected, gangrenous, root-canaled tooth, all in a misguided attempt to make the tooth "stronger!" Do not let the natural appearance of a crown fool you into believing it is a good procedure for the tooth. A crown is a cruel illusion of an ideal tooth. Underneath the crown lies the stub of the tooth- -all that is left after the dentist prepares it to hold the crown.

Dentists Who Specialize In Crowns

Dentists are taught to believe that the crown specialists are the elite of the profession; they do the fancy work and get the high fees. Indeed, this kind of dental work does require a high level of skill. The fanciest work is done when a patient has only a few teeth left in one arch. If the teeth are spread around the arch, the specialist will make a horseshoe-shaped bridge that fits a crown on each of the teeth left (or on an implant) and place a false tooth in all the spaces. This horseshoe bridge is then cemented to the teeth. This horseshoe-shaped, full arch bridge is considered a spectacular example of the dental arts and looks like a perfect set of teeth. However, to call it "Hollywood dentistry" is more appropriate because the result is more illusion than reality. The reality can be seen in the X-rays. The teeth, commonly treated with root-canals, have weak bone support, abscesses, and gum problems. Thus these bridges rarely last long because the remaining teeth are asked to do the work of a full set of natural teeth.

What happens when one of these teeth fail? The whole horseshoe bridge fails. At $800 to $1000 per tooth or more, the bridge is a substantial "investment." But this "investment in health," as it is sometimes called, may actually result in "dental bankruptcy" as the bridge's support fails. While these bridges are often written about in dental journals, they are seldom-mentioned 5 years later.

As long as dentists think they can duplicate and even improve on nature, the emphasis will be on repairing, rather than preventing, disease. Until dentists are seriously willing to take on the real causes of dental problems, sugar addiction and poor nutrition, nothing will improve and the dental profession will continue to be repair-oriented "tooth mechanics."

Crowns

Crowning a tooth means reshaping the tooth by removing part of the enamel and dentin and then covering it with a strong dental material, usually metal. A crown can also be used individually or as part of a fixed (cemented) bridge that replaces a missing tooth. Among dentists, doing crowns is considered the key to building a successful practice. The number of crowns done per week is commonly used to judge how well a practice is being managed.

The key way that the need for a crown is "presented" (dental term for selling) to the patient is that "it is necessary to crown this weak tooth to save it." But regardless of what your dentist might tell you about the need to crown badly damaged teeth to "save" them, the opposite is much more likely, that is, crowning always makes the tooth weaker. For many teeth crowning leads to death of the nerve and eventual loss.

Preparing The Tooth

The destruction of the tooth begins in preparing it for the crown as the dentist reshapes the tooth using a diamond-covered bur. These burs come in different grits from coarse (which can cut the tooth very quickly) to very fine and in different shapes and sizes. Some dentists have boasted that they can cut down a tooth for a crown in 90 seconds. Unfortunately, rapidly cutting diamond burs can bum the tooth because of friction. More importantly, cutting down a tooth for a crown removes a large portion of the tooth structure, including virtually all of the enamel.

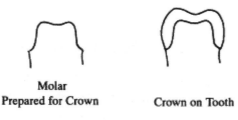

Molar
Prepared for Crown   Crown on Tooth

Molar

Figure 11.1

Since the amount of tooth structure that must be removed is similar whether the crown is being made for a large or a small tooth, a higher percentage of the tooth structure is removed from the smaller teeth. Unfortunately, many of these small teeth do not

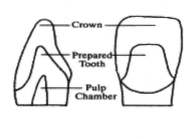

Side View   Front View

Central Incisor

Figure 11.2

have much tooth structure in the first place. Front teeth, particularly the lower front teeth, are much smaller than molars, requiring a greater percentage of their enamel and dentin to be removed than from a molar. It is common to have a front tooth die after being crowned, because so little tooth structure is left to protect the nerve chamber.

Why Is The Enamel Removed?

Why would a dentist destroy the enamel--the tooth's most valuable protective tissue? Dentists do not like having to remove all the enamel, but they must to make the crown fit. The actual crown is made outside of the mouth, so the shaping of the tooth is necessary for the crown to be made in the dental lab and then to fit back on the tooth.

Most dentists do not stop to consider the procedures and materials used in the crowning; they are so well indoctrinated while in school that they never question whether crowning is really a good idea. Why are they taught this way? The procedures used to crown teeth have been developed not to protect the tooth, but to fit the needs of the materials and the lab techniques.

Materials Used For Crowns

The materials used to crown teeth may be biocompatible, but are more often a threat to the immune system and to the survival of the tooth itself. Some materials, such as porcelain, require much more tooth structure to be removed, because they need to be thicker for strength. (Not the tooth's strength, but the crown's strength.) That removal makes the tooth weaker and more prone to dying. To make matters worse, most dentists see nothing wrong in leaving pieces of the old mercury fillings under the crowns. That's a double whammy!

The hardness of the metals and the roughness of the porcelains create a problem in getting the bite right. It is common for crowns to damage opposing teeth on their biting (occlusal) surface, causing the non-crowned tooth to become sensitive or even killing it. It has been suggested recently that crowns should be replaced every 10 years to adjust for the natural wear of the teeth. In other words, the materials used for crowns are too hard for natural wearing.

In order to fit the hard materials used in a crown onto the tooth, it must be reduced in size and changed in shape. The farther down the root the crown preparation goes, the more of the tooth must be removed. Thus, the tooth tissue is removed to make the technique work, not to help the tooth. Yet it is plain to see that cutting away tooth structure can never be better for the tooth; it always weakens it.

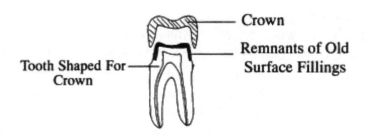

Crown Over Old Mercury Filling

Figure 11.3

The "Crack In The Tooth" Sales Pitch

Many dentists cannot resist the urge to crown every possible tooth. It is common to hear a patient say the reason the dentist crowned his tooth is because it had a "crack" in it. Teeth do get cracks in them, but this is not a valid reason to grind off all the enamel. The cracks rarely cause a problem, and if a piece of enamel were to come off, the area could easily be repaired with a bonded composite. In fact, if a dentist is worried about a crack, he can bond over it to give the enamel more strength, rather than removing the enamel by grinding it away. It is quite possible that the majority of cracks in teeth are caused by the expansion of the mercury fillings, which means that dentists caused cracks in the first place.

Crowning Weakens Teeth

Remember, the tooth and the crown are two different structures. The metal crown covering the tooth must be strong because it has to compensate for the dentist-caused weak tooth. If a tooth was weak before crowning, it will be much weaker afterward. However, it is not necessary for a dentist to grind off all the enamel to restore a damaged tooth.

The new bondable composite materials can rebuild a tooth no matter what shape the damage has taken, because composites are moldable to any shape. Thus, composite bonding techniques do not require any undamaged tooth structure to be removed. In fact, this technique must be conservative because it needs every bit of natural tooth structure possible on which to bond.

To understand the difference between restoring a tooth with composite and covering it with a crown, consider the following analogy. If you have a home whose siding needs to be painted often, you may wish to cover it with vinyl siding, a thin layer of material that covers and protects the wood. Before the wood is covered, any damaged or decayed boards can be repaired. The vinyl is then added strip by strip over the wood. That is the same method used when composites are added to a damaged or decayed tooth. Only the bad parts are removed; the rest is protected by a carefully applied covering of composite.

In contrast, to "crown" a house you would have to remove all the clapboard and part of the underlying supporting studs and beams before a solid covering could be lowered over and cemented to the whole house at once. In removing so much of the structure of the house to allow the covering to fit in one piece, structural damage may occur that could destroy vital systems. And once this one-piece covering is in place, you could not see out of the windows and no air or moisture could escape; it would be sealed.

A crown does the same to the tooth. Vital tissues are removed and a hard structure is placed as a covering over the remains of the tooth, sealing it. Since crowning is very destructive to a tooth. And since you have other options, there is no longer any justification for using this technique. The tooth cannot speak for itself. As a patient, you must say, "No!" to crowns.

Selling Crowns

Although dentists earn a good deal of their income from crowns and bridges, not one dentist will admit to placing a crown on a tooth just for the extra income. Dentists cannot deny that all the practice management seminars tell them they must "do more crowns to increase practice profitability." Since most dental practices would not survive economically without doing crowns, there will be much resistance to stopping the use of these techniques. Many dentists have quota systems as to how many crowns must be "sold" each week and month, with staff members sharing in the profits.

Insurance companies are partly to blame for the profit motive in using crowns. The dentist may suggest that since the patient has insurance, it will not cost him very much to have the "best dentistry has to offer." Actually, many patients have the crown done only because the insurance pays for part of it. Without insurance, they would probably have nothing done. This type of overuse of insurance for elective procedures is behind the huge increase of all medical costs. Remember, Blue Cross/Blue Shield was set up by doctors in the first place. After all, being self-serving is the name of the game. The plans are sold as a benefit, but it seems that the insurance companies and the dentists benefit most.

Dentists Believe In Crowns

Dentists will tell you that they crown teeth because they "believe" that the tooth will benefit from the procedure. They use the reasons they were taught in dental school by dentists who also learned these reasons in dental school. They are taught that crowns make the tooth stronger, can correct the position, the bite, the shape, and the appearance of the tooth. In truth, crowning a tooth can have the opposite effects, making the tooth weaker, be incorrectly positioned, ruin the bite, be wrongly shaped, and appear phony.

Even if all those reasons had been at one time valid, there are now safer, more conservative ways to fix teeth by using bonding composite materials. Unfortunately, dentists will be slow to adopt the new materials to replace crowns for a number of reasons. They will say that the new materials are not "strong enough." Although these materials may not be as strong as metal, they are strong enough. This criticism is common as dentists are always underestimating the strength of composites. Just as composite fillings properly done can outlast mercury fillings, they may also outlast many crowns. In addition, unlike crowns, they are far less expensive and may be repaired if damaged or if further decay happens. (The tooth that remains under the crown can still decay.) Composites are easier on the tooth, on the patient, and on the wallet.

An Option To Crowning

If dentists are uncomfortable placing a large composite instead of a crown because they feel it is too "technique-sensitive," they have another option. Instead of crowns, dentists can use lab-made composite inlays and onlays. If 80 percent of a tooth's enamel is already gone, a large onlay can be made that will save the remaining enamel versus crowning, which would remove it. If 20 percent is all the enamel left, it becomes very important to save it and not to think that since so much is already gone, what is a little bit more!

Inlays and onlays are bonded onto the tooth, so it is not necessary to drastically reshape the tooth as is done with a crown, although inlays and onlays do require more removal of tooth structure than for a composite filling. Dentists know that

307

these are great restorations and can easily replace crowns, but they do not routinely use the new materials in this way. Again, this may be because they rely too much on their earlier training and experience. It is time for them to retrain and gain new experience.

Eventually, dentists may understand that they have been misled by their training to believe crowning a tooth is good for a tooth. But when they think about it, the truth of what is done to a tooth to make a crown is just too terrible to continue using this procedure. Dentists may think that if they change the way they practice, patients may blame them for problems brought on by the crowns they made before. To make it easy for them, let us say from this day forth, there is no more need to crown teeth; that way, dentists need not be defensive about teeth that they have already crowned.

Crowning Can Kill Teeth

As you can see, there are many reasons not to have a crown made, but the biggest reason is: CROWNING TEETH CAN KILL THEM. The ADA admits that on the average, one crowned tooth in five—20 percent—will die. This percentage varies from dentist to dentist. Some dentists are skilled and will cause only a very few teeth to die, while others may kill almost every tooth they crown.

If you asked a dentist what percentage of the teeth he has crowned died within 5 years, he will be unable to answer. Dentists neither keep such records, nor think in those terms. Dentists probably do not "believe" they kill any teeth. When one dies, they believe that it "just happened." Some teeth die quickly, while others may take years. In either case, a dying tooth makes life miserable for the patient with its chronic aching and hot and cold sensitivity.

Rationalizing Post-Crowning Damage

How do dentists view the damage done by the crowning procedure? They do not consider a dying tooth as a major problem because they think they can just do a root-canal and "save" it. Once a patient pays $600 for a crown, he will agree to whatever procedure the dentist tells him is necessary to "save" the tooth, even if it costs another $500. Unfortunately, a root-canal is a terrible burden on the immune system and should also be avoided. (See "ROOT-CANALS.")

Since many dentists believe that a crowned tooth dies because it was weak to begin with, they may even recommend doing a root-canal before crowning to "prevent problems." That is a scary thought, but not unusual. These dentists know that doing a root-canal after a crown is made is more difficult and leaves a hole in the crown. Doing the root-canal first they believe they are making the tooth more "trouble-free." Ironically, every time dentists do something they "believe" is making the tooth stronger, they are really weakening it.

Dentists know that crowning teeth damages the teeth because they are taught not to crown a tooth until a person reaches his twenties because the pulp chamber (which contains the tooth's vital tissues, including the nerve) is large in young people and crowning will damage it. But as the tooth matures, it becomes smaller, so by the patient's mid-twenties, dentists are taught that it is okay to cut the tooth down for a crown. If damage is possible in an immature tooth, it is possible in a mature one only at a reduced level.

Longevity of Crowns

The final reason not to crown a tooth is the concept of "What happens next?" A crown does not last forever, may fail in as little as a year or may last 40 years without major problems. But if a crown only lasts an average of 15 to 20 years, you must ask the question "What happens next?" It is uncommon for a dentist to redo a crown; more of the tooth would have to be removed, increasing the chances for side effects. It is more likely that a crowned tooth would be extracted for a reason probably directly related to its being crowned in the first place.

Recommendation: If a tooth does not have a crown on it, do not have one made. At this time, there is no valid reason to crown a tooth and many reasons to avoid doing it. Any large restorations can be done with an inlay or onlay.

Measuring The Loss of Tooth Structure

When a tooth is prepared for a crown, a certain amount of tooth structure must be removed. For most crowning materials, a minimum of one millimeter must be removed from each side, including the top, and in many areas a millimeter and a half is removed. That may not sound like much, but must be viewed in relation to the size of the tooth.

An average molar is approximately 10 X 11 X 6 millimeters. When you multiply length times width times height, you get the volume of the part of the tooth that we see in the mouth. In this example the numbers equal 660 cubic millimeters. Now if the tooth is prepared for a crown, and one millimeter is removed from each side, the new dimensions would be 8 X 9 X 5 or 360 cubic millimeters. The molar has been reduced 45 percent, a reduction of almost half of its volume. If a millimeter and a half

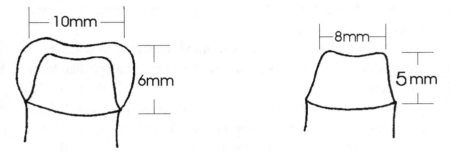

Tooth Before Preparation   **Tooth After Preparation**

Figure 11.4

were removed, the volume would be 7 X 8 X 4.5, which leaves only 252 cubic millimeters, or a 62 percent reduction. That means the crowning procedure left only 38 percent of the tooth structure above the gums; a shocking amount of reduction.

These percentages show what happens to a molar, but consider the loss in crowning other teeth, which are smaller in volume. The crowning procedure requires the same shaping to be done on any tooth, so the same amount of tooth structure, one millimeter to one and a half millimeters on every side, must be removed, no matter what tooth is being crowned. A bicuspid is half the size of a molar, approximately 5 X 10 X 6 or 300 cubic millimeters. Cutting off one millimeter would reduce the volume to 3 X 8 x 5, leaving only 120 cubic millimeters or 40 percent of the tooth. An upper front tooth is even smaller and has a tapering shape that makes computing the amount of reduction difficult.

Preparing an upper front tooth for a crown would involve at least a 60 percent reduction. The smallest teeth are the four lower front teeth. After they are cut down to be crowned, they look like toothpicks, and it is quite possible that only 25 percent of the tooth is left. And remember, inside the remains of the tooth (many patients call it a "stump") is the pulp chamber, even in the tiny remnants of these lower front teeth.

With these measurements in mind, it is easy to understand how damaging the crowning procedure is. Do not forget that teeth are organs. In essence, crowning means removing 40 to 75 percent of an organ just to cover the tooth with a metal or porcelain shell. How many organs would not be badly damaged or even destroyed if a similar treatment were done to them? Although the ADA reports that 20 percent of teeth die as a result of crowning, it is surprising that any of them survive such a brutal procedure. The worse part is that most, if not all, crowns need not be done.

Large Filling Rationale

Dentists will make the argument that many teeth they select to crown already have large fillings, so much of the tooth structure has already been removed in doing the filling. While this may seem a reasonable rationale, it is really strengthening the argument against crowning. For example, a tooth has already had 50 percent of its enamel removed for a filling, shaping for a crown would just remove the remaining 50 percent. The attitude should be "that poor tooth's already lost 50 percent of its enamel, so we must do everything possible to protect the enamel that's left!" The more enamel that has already been removed, then the more important it is to save the enamel that remains. Fortunately, dentists have techniques available, direct bonded composites and bonded composite inlays and onlays, that can strengthen and protect the tooth while retaining remaining enamel. There is no need to destroy the tooth to "save" it.

Replacing Crowns

If you already have crowns, you need to thoroughly understand your options. In a perfect world, your dentist would be able to remove the old crown, remove all the old metal, and place a new, non-metal crown. New materials available since 1997 make a non-metal crown possible. The following list of crowning materials will give you an idea of the problems possible with each kind.

Enamel Rating: 5 to 0. The rating on remaking any crown is based on the damage done during the initial preparation of the tooth. Once the enamel is removed, it cannot be replaced. When a tooth is reprepared for another crown, even more tooth structure must be removed.

Crowning Materials

Porcelain: Besides the metal factor in porcelain, it is also brittle and glass-like, so it does break, chip, and fracture. To help prevent this breakage, the tooth must be cut down even more than what is done for a metal or porcelain-over-metal crown. This deeper cut allows for a thicker porcelain covering strong enough to keep from breaking under normal use. However, this deeper cutting also reduces the amount of the original tooth that is left and therefore, increases the chance of the tooth dying.

Gold: Many dentists who practice mercury-free dentistry use a lot of gold to replace fillings, instead of using composite. If you are going to use this material, the gold content should be very high. There are few golds that do not have many other metals added. You must be careful. A material compatibility study may help you find a gold you can tolerate, but remember, it is highly possible that a compatibility test done while you have a lot of mercury and other metals in your mouth may not be accurate. Another possibility to keep in mind is that you can become intolerant of any metal placed in your mouth, even gold, after having it for a few years.

Furthermore, like all metals, gold generates electric currents in your mouth, sometimes causing some very high electrical readings. If a dentist places a gold crown over part of a mercury filling, which is routinely done, an especially strong electrical field is created within the tooth. It is common for this electric current to weaken the tooth so much that decay begins at the gum line. The odds are that over one-half of all crowns on the back teeth have mercury under them.

Not surprisingly, dentists tend to do the more expensive procedures first, so replacing crowns or doing new ones before all the mercury has been removed can often happen. However, this should NEVER be done. Gold attracts mercury. The mercury from the old fillings will contaminate the new gold dental work. You may end up no better off than you were before.

Composite: Composite crowns, which are made of the same material as composite fillings, can be made by a dental lab. Their biggest advantage over composites done directly on the tooth is that shrinkage problems are minimized when the crown is bonded to the tooth. No information on longevity is available, since this is a new technique, but the average life span is probably close to 10 years. If you test compatible to composite fillings, then this is a good option, as it means all the material used in your mouth will be the same, reducing the chances for sensitivity.

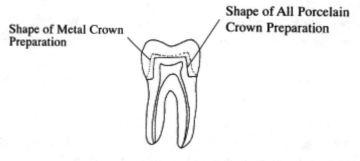

Tooth Structure Removed For Porcelain Crown

Figure 11.5

Acrylic: Acrylic material may be used for temporary crowns, but usually lasts only 6 to 18 months before chewing wears them down.

Titanium: Of the other metals available, titanium may be suggested to you as the most biocompatible, but presents many problems. First, pure titanium would have to be used which makes it very difficult--almost impossible--to work with. Second, titanium is a shiny, silvery-looking metal that is quite unattractive. Third, due to its hardness, the bite is almost impossible to get right. And finally, titanium carries and generates electrical charges, and its use is better avoided.

Palladium, a "semi-precious" metal, is commonly used. Like titanium, it is better to avoid unless recommended on your compatibility test. The same is true of the dozens of new alloys that contain numerous other metals.

Nickel: The worst metal is nickel because it is carcinogenic (cancer-causing). In addition, it causes hypersensitive reactions in one percent of men and 10 percent of women, yet it is used in millions of crowns because it is the cheapest alloy. It has been estimated that currently 70 percent of crowns are nickel. Just think how many crowns you could make out of one stainless steel pot--hundreds! That's right; stainless steel contains a high percentage of nickel and chromium, both carcinogens. Your stainless steel cookware adds some of these metals to any food cooked in it. Thus, using stainless steel cookware should also be avoided. Like mercury fillings, nickel crowns should be immediately banned by the FDA.

The Use of Radioactive Metals

The March 2000 Bio-Probe Newsletter reported that a Swedish researcher, Ulf Bengtsson, has found 35 references to radioactive materials used as dental materials. The manufacturers do not state that such materials are used in their products but it is allowed under current FDA standards. The only way to find if a radioactive material is indeed in a product is to do a chemical analysis. Its use had been limited to porcelains to make it more lifelike. Does this make sense to you? Does using radioactive materials in people's mouths to make teeth look lifelike and in the process possibly killing them make sense to you? This should not be allowed and the only thing you can do is shake your head in amazement

It is bad enough that radioactive material is in some porcelains, but it is now possible to find it in composites, too, used to make fillings show up on X-rays better than just using metal in the glass fillers because it is denser. He lists the proposed metal fillers in composites including uranium, thorium, lead, mercury, barium, bismuth, and zirconium.

Is your head shaking yet? It should be. Are you confused, thinking that you might as well leave the mercury fillings in rather than switching to radioactive metals? There are ways you can avoid these materials. First, use no porcelains. Even if the dentist swears there are no radioactive metals used, there is no way the dentist can be sure he is right. No one tells the dentists. The only way you can be sure that the composite used in your teeth is that it does not show up on X-rays. This is quite certain way to check, as metal-free composite fillers do not show up on X-rays

The use of radioactive luminous dials on watches has been banned but now it seems okay to put into your teeth. This is a sorry day, but there is no evidence that it causes cancer in people. Well, it might, but since no studies have been done, no one knows. Radioactive material's purpose in porcelain is to give it natural luminescence. "Sorry, your husband died, but don't his teeth look great?…not only now but when someone digs him up in ten thousand years, his teeth will still look good!"

As mentioned, the material used in our office is Visiofil which does not show up on X-rays because there are no metals in it. Radioactive metals may already be in some materials, and there is no way to tell from the information the companies give out. The burden is on the dentists and the patients. It is scandalous! The

ADA brags about using mercury for 150 years, about fluoridating your water, about using nickel in most crowns, braces and partials, and now radioactive metals. You can only shake your head in amazement at the anti-health attitude of "modern" dentistry.

Information on safe materials is critical for patients, but you cannot rely on old information. Information needs to be continuously updated. I urge you to check our website (**dentistry-toothtruth.com**) for any new information before you have any work done. It is hoped that there will be new, safer materials developed, perhaps a baseless hope, as the materials seem to be getting more dangerous. The old rule applies: The simpler the better. It seems that dentistry is antagonistic to the normal physiology of the human body. Arthur L. Kraslow, M.D., once said, *"The individual has the right of his wisdom to choose methods for his well being and longevity. This right is not to be taken from us."* Do not let your dentist take this right from you.

Ruined Health Is Not A Bargain

Although many patients are rightly concerned about how long the crown will last, the more important question is, "Can the material in any way hurt my health?" It is best to guide your decision by how it may affect you, because a crown that can last for the rest of your life but ruins your health is not a bargain. Biocompatibility is always the first consideration.

Composite is a safe material for the vast majority of dental patients. At this point, the biggest risk may be financial. For instance, if you use a less strong composite crown over a gold one and it breaks, you will need to replace it, but removing the health risks of having toxic, or potentially toxic, metals in your body may be well worth it. Besides, failures can happen with any of the materials, even gold.

The greatest source of failure with crowns will be from the damage done to the tooth by the crowning procedure or the inaccurate shape or fit of the crown and not by the material breaking. One way to add to the strength of a composite crown is to bond it onto the tooth using the new bonding cements which give greater support than regular cements. This technique may add years to the crown's life.

Reducing Costs of Remaking Crowns

There is one way you can reduce the cost in case the crown breaks and must be remade. When you have a crown made, ask your dentist for the models that the dental lab used to make it. (You need to ask in advance as they are usually discarded after the crown is cemented.) A new crown can be made from these models that will fit as well as the first one; this should reduce replacement costs to only a lab fee plus a cementing fee. One-third to one-half of the current fee for a crown would be reasonable.

Placing a composite crown may become a popular option with dentists because it is very close to the technique used for metal crowns. The fee would be the same. Doing composite crowns would allow the dentists to maintain a key financial part of their practice.

Do Not Be In A Hurry

If you want to be metal-free and your dentist cannot or will not do non-metal crowns, wait until you find someone who can. Be conservative; do not be in a hurry. It is your mouth and your money, so get what you need and nothing less. Do not be intimidated by the "you are the patient and I am the doctor" attitude. You know more about yourself than anyone else.

New, more biocompatibile materials for crowns may eventually become available. Any replacement materials used now to get the metals out of your body can be replaced then.

Dental Bridges

Bridges are two or more crowns connected, with at least one of the two replacing a missing tooth. The most common configuration is a three-tooth bridge with a crown on either side of the missing tooth. The problems found in single crowns are multiplied when doing a bridge. If it is a bad idea to remove half a tooth's structure to make a crown, it is a worse idea to remove half of the tooth structure of two teeth to replace one missing tooth. Even worse is that often one or both of the teeth next to the missing tooth will not even have fillings, which makes it doubly wrong since it becomes necessary to cut down perfect teeth to make a bridge.

Besides the permanent damage done to a tooth preparing it for a crown, bridges cause other problems. It has been the rule that to make a bridge strong, it had to be made with metal. With the new materials, non-metal bridges can now be made. The use of metals can cause an immune system reaction or there may be reactions to the electricity the metals generate. Problems can also occur with getting and keeping the occlusion correct. In addition, the longevity of a bridge is usually shorter than the patient's life span, necessitating further more elaborate treatment in the future. Finally, the patient faces the strong possibility that one of the crowned teeth will die. These negatives far outweigh any advantages a bridge may have for the patient.

It is now possible to make bridges from composite materials reinforced with Kevlar fibers. These fibers are strong and give an option not available before 1997. Using conservative inlay preparations on the abutment teeth, a bridge that is kinder to healthy teeth can be done without the destruction of full crowns.

Enamel rating: 0 Bridges get the lowest rating of all procedures because the enamel is removed from two or more sometimes-perfect teeth to create the shape necessary for them to fit. This technique is the most destructive of any dental procedure.

Replacing An Existing Bridge

Replacing an existing bridge is one of the most difficult challenges facing a patient who wants to be metal-free. The damage done when the bridge was made makes it almost impossible to get a good result. Crowning teeth limits future possible options. A bridge can be replaced with a composite bridge, the simplest option if you want to be metal-free.

Replacing A Missing Tooth

Tens of millions of Americans are missing one or more back teeth. Of the several treatment options each has negative consequences. There is a greater possibility of causing more damage by replacing the missing tooth than if nothing were done, and the risks increase as the treatments become more elaborate. In addition, as the treatments become more elaborate, the options for alternative treatments become fewer and the probability of negative side effects become greater.

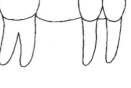

Missing Tooth

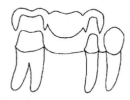

Teeth Prepared for Bridge
Cross-Section

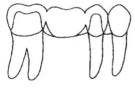

Bridge In Place

Dental Bridges

Figure 11.6

Available Options

To illustrate how the "risks versus benefits" concept applies in this case, assume you are missing a lower first molar. You have four options from which to choose: 1) Do nothing; 2) make a one-tooth removable partial; 3) make a "fixed" bridge; or 4) have an implant placed in the bone and a replacement crown put on top.

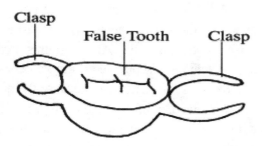

One Tooth Removable Partial

One Tooth Removable Partial

Figure 11.7

The following are options and their possible consequences:

1) Do nothing: If nothing is done, over many years (10 or more) the neighboring and opposing teeth will move into the space, causing areas difficult to clean that could lead to decay and/or gum problems. A missing tooth also lowers the chewing efficiency on that side, although most patients who "do nothing" do not seem to notice. These people are reluctant to try the other options because they feel they are doing very well without the tooth. You may be surprised to know that this is the option most people choose. Remember, that "doing nothing" is always an option because almost all dental procedures are elective, meaning that you can choose to follow the dentist's recommendation or not.

Enamel rating: No change.

2) Removable Partial: A one-tooth removable partial is a false tooth that can be put in and taken out. (See Fig. 9.6) The partial stays in place by holding onto the neighboring teeth with arms called "clasps."

It is possible to have two teeth on these partials but more than that may stress the clasped teeth. These partials are called "unilateral" or one-sided partials. Although this treatment is a viable option, it is actively discouraged during a dentist's training. The instructors may feel it is dangerous because the partial is small enough to be swallowed, while possible, it is not likely. It is possible that the teachers were taught not to make one-tooth partials when they were students and never challenged their teaching. Therefore, the negative attitude toward these unilateral partials is perpetuated.

While unilateral partials may be made from metal, they can be made without metal by using Flexite, a good non-metal replacement option because even the clasps can be made with Flexite. Thus, it is as safe an option as "doing nothing."

If the partial breaks, it is repairable; if it wears out, it can be replaced for a few hundred dollars. If anything happens to the teeth that are clasped, they can be fixed and the partial should still fit. The partial can be replaced over and over without any additional work being done to the teeth. One slight drawback is that these partials must be removed during tooth brushing because it is essential that the surrounding teeth be kept very clean. Partials should not be worn at night.

Enamel rating: no change.

3) Fixed bridge: A fixed bridge requires that the teeth on either side of the space be shaped to hold a crown, inlay or onlay. After the bridge is made, it is cemented or bonded (fixed) to the prepared teeth. This procedure is hard on teeth and may eventually cause them to die, as with any crowned tooth. If inlays or onlays preparations are used, chances that the tooth will die from the procedure are much less than with a crown preparation. Let us assume the following: the teeth do not die, although the odds may be as high as two chances in five that one of the two teeth dies if the teeth are crowned; it is made from the most biocompatible gold, porcelain or composite; it is made to fit the prepared teeth perfectly and is cemented correctly; and the crowns are perfectly shaped, with no over-contouring or under-contouring, which could cause gum problems. (Studies show that the gums are more likely to be swollen and bleed around a crown than around a natural tooth.)

More Problems

Given all these assumptions of perfection, what else could happen? If any old mercury filling is left under the crown, an electrical current could be set up that promotes decay. Metal used will create some electric current. Another possible source of problems is the bite. Even if the crown were made perfectly, which is difficult, the normal bite changes over the years. Because the crowning materials are hard except composite crowns or inlays, they resist wear, which means the opposing natural teeth get double wear. Also, any change in the bite that puts more pressure on the tooth can lead to bone damage, which can seriously weaken the bridge. A common problem is that the patient does not clean the bridge well, particularly under the false tooth; this can cause swollen gums, breakdown of the bone support, and/or decay at the edge of the crown.

Bridges are estimated to last more than 10 years and some last more than 20 years. But they can also fail very quickly if not done well or if the supporting teeth are too weak. If 20 years is assumed for our example, then the question must be asked, "What happens next?" If the patient was 30 when the bridge was placed, then at age 50 he will need something else to be done. Another bridge is possible, if there has not been too much damage. Another consideration is the cost of a bridge, which can be five times the cost of Option 2, a removable partial. In other words, you could have five removable bridges made for the cost of one fixed bridge. (Dentists like to call them permanent bridges," but they are not really permanent.)

If a second bridge can be made, it will probably not last as long as the first, because more damage has been done to the supporting gums and bone over the years. But let's assume the patient is lucky and it lasts 15 years. The patient is now 65 with another 10 or 20 more years left to live.

What's the next option, a third bridge? Possible, but highly unlikely. After 35 years, most dentists would expect that one of the crowned teeth would be lost, making a cemented bridge less likely or impossible. Other teeth may have been lost by now. All the teeth may have gum problems, and they may all need extracting. So at best, 25 to 35 years would be all that one could hope for from fixed bridges.

If all bridges did as well as this example, choosing this option might not be a bad idea. But in our example, we assumed that many common problems were avoided. In reality, these are common areas of failure and a great number of bridges fail if one or more of these problems exist. A fair number of bridges fail before 10 years leaving a larger problem than the original missing tooth.

If only perfect patients were selected, then the example might be a good average, but dentists tend to put bridges in any patients that will agree to pay for them. The reality is that the average life span of all bridges is closer to 15 to 20 years, and few of the teeth crowned to make the bridge are healthy enough after 20 years to hold a second bridge. That means the average patient would have to face a more serious problem in their 40's or 50's caused by the failure of the bridge.

The worse problem would be if any of the teeth died and root canals were done. Crowned teeth abscessing is common and may be deadly. Any procedure that can cause a tooth to die should be avoided.

Enamel rating: 0. This is worse than doing a single crown because more than one tooth is having its enamel removed. In addition, the teeth that happen to be next to the open space usually do not meet the criteria dentists use to recommend crowns so these unfortunate teeth are being severely damaged just to do the bridge.

4) An Implant:
Implants "represent an outstanding business opportunity."
Cheryl Farr, *Dentistry Today*, June 1994

The technique for doing an implant is much more difficult than for a bridge and takes much longer than people expect. A hole must be made in the bone, the implant put in the hole, and the gums sewn closed, covering the implant while the bone grows around and onto it. After sufficient healing an opening is made to the implant and a post is screwed into it. On the post is placed whatever is needed, in this case a crown. Let us assume that all the above steps go flawlessly and that the crown fits the implant post perfectly and is cemented correctly.

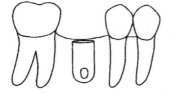 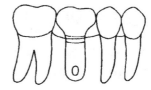

Implant In Bone   **Implant With Crown**

Implants

Figure 11.8

Even if the procedure were done perfectly, and that is a big assumption, other problems can occur because there is a major difference between a tooth and an implant. A tooth is attached to the bone by tiny ligaments which act as shock absorbers, letting you sense the hardness of what you are chewing, while an implant is coated so that the bone attaches directly to it, making the bite extremely critical. If too heavy the implant could be damaged or lost, if it is too light, you cannot chew well. Another major difference between an implant and a real tooth is that the gums are not attached to the implant but only "snug up" to the collar that surrounds the post where it comes through the gums, leaving an opening from the mouth down the side of the post to the bone. Bacteria can make this trip easily, particularly if the oral hygiene is less than perfect. To make matters much worse, the collar is usually made of nickel, a cancer-causing metal or titanium, and all of these metals create electrical current, which is grounded into the bone like a lightning rod. Implants may trigger autoimmune problems.

If a single missing tooth is being replaced with an implant, the crown that fits on the implant must fit perfectly in the space between the other two teeth; if it is too tight, it will not go in, so can only be the perfect size or too small. If too small, then food will tend to pack between the teeth and the implant's crown, causing damage to the gums and quickly damaging the implant or adjacent tooth.

Maintaining Healthy Tissues

If you choose the implant option, remember that keeping the false tooth and the gums around it perfectly clean is the most critical part of maintaining the implant. If the original tooth was lost due to gum disease, then an implant is a bad idea, because the dietary problems that caused the tooth to be lost in the first place will work against the survivability of the implant. Even for relatively healthy individuals, the nutritional needs for maintaining healthy bone are very important. Extra attention may be needed in areas of diet and mineral supplementation, but these areas are probably not discussed by the majority of dentists who place implants. "Eat a balanced diet" might be the only nutritional advice the implant patient receives. Osteoporosis, a real threat to the survival of both teeth and implants, means white, post-menopausal women are generally bad candidates for this option.

Another potential problem with implants to keep in mind is that some popular brands need to have the crown removed every year and a new "shock absorbing" insert placed in the implant, adding over a hundred dollars in maintenance costs each year. The insert is held in place with a screw that has a tendency to get loose, but if over-tightened, its threads can be stripped--a disaster because the threads are in the actual implant and it may be difficult or impossible to repair. If this disaster happens, it may be possible to re-thread the implant. If the repair fails the implant must be removed altogether and replaced or abandoned and left in the bone. Either of these options has many problems, such as contamination of the bone with metal fragments if the implant is cut out or open access to the bone for oral bacteria if it is left. In addition, potential comfort problems can arise in trying to find a functional treatment when there is an abandoned implant underneath.

Longevity

How long will an implant last? Dentists who place implants say that over 90 percent last 10 years or more. The question then must be asked, "What happens next?" A second implant is rare because whatever causes the first to be lost would stop a new one from being placed. Basically, you can only get one implant at each acceptable site. If the patient was 35 when the implant was placed, he may only be 45 when it fails. If it lasted 20 years, he would only be 55. In either case, no further treatment may be the only treatment possible.

Another source of trouble with a failed implant is that it could damage any natural teeth next to it, a particular problem when used to replace a single missing front tooth on a relatively young person. Many dentists who place implants use them for single teeth because it is the easiest type of implant placement. Using single-tooth implants is the most common type even though the ADA recommends against such usage. The ADA would recommend Option 3, a fixed bridge, more than any other for many reasons, most having nothing to do with the patient.

High Cost

The cost for an implant is greater than a fixed bridge (Option 3), not even including the cost of the yearly maintenance and the risk of a short life span. Fortunately, because of the high costs, implants are still not being commonly done, but their use is growing and they are being promoted as one of the key ways to make a dental practice grow. But, with all their problems, implants should be considered experimental at best. Implants would be too expensive if they were free. A prudent attitude should be, "Let the dentists experiment on other people."

Dental Attitudes

Dentists may refuse to treat you if you do not want to do what they recommend. However, if you tell them up front that you want to go by the concepts in this book, then their egos may not get involved. They may think you are crazy or misdirected, but they may do it your way merely to see what happens. They may even ask you to sign a paper stating that the treatments were done at your insistence. Use your own judgment. Signing a paper neither excuses incompetence nor means you have waived any legal rights, only that you were aware of any problems before treatment began.

You will be better off if you can find a dentist with a lot of experience in doing composites, a search that may temporarily become difficult, as more and more patients want their metal fillings removed. In the near future, dentists who know how to remove metal property will be fully booked. Then, as other dentists see the trend, more and more will learn the proper procedures until the supply of trained dentists catches up with the demand. It is important that only dentists trained in proper removal techniques do the work, because if removal is done improperly, a person could get sicker. The International Association of Oral Medicine and Toxicology (IAOMT) have developed a certification process so that dentists with the proper training can be identified by the public. Log onto the internet at www.IAOMT.org.

How Sick Are You?

For the very sick person it is important to get the work done as soon as possible to avoid being trapped by fully booked dentists. Remember, if every person who has work to be done were treated and all the dentists worked at it full time, it would take 5 to 10 years to completely remove the toxic metals from people's mouths. Each person must decide if his health can afford to wait that long.

Conclusion

It is difficult for people to think 10 years into the future. If our cars last longer than the payments, we are happy. If a dentist tells a patient that a dental bridge will last 10 to 20 years, the patient will think that is a long time, but it really is not. The question, "What happens next?" needs to be routinely asked.

You may be surprised that dentists do not think in terms of "What happens next?" They, too, think 10 or 20 years is a long time for a dental treatment to last. They may figure that they are doing the best they can, and when their last treatment fails, they will find a new treatment. They simply do not consider how one treatment often requires an additional treatment later on. This failure to look ahead is why the "guided destruction of the teeth" is the best way to describe the reality of the current practice of dentistry.

These four options for dealing with a missing tooth give you an idea of how you must think when a dentist suggests treatment for you. When you consider any of the options, you must think in terms of your lifetime, not any shorter time span. You must have an idea of how long the proposed treatment will last and what you will need after that treatment fails, and keep thinking of how you can maintain the teeth you have now for the rest of your life. Most treatment plans eventually lead to a dead end with nothing left to do but endure. An unspoken hope exists among dentists that when patients run out of dental treatment options, they will die, so dentists do not have to face the patient with the truth that after a lifetime of "care," no treatments remain to help them.

When seeking treatment for yourself and your family rely on what you have learned here. Do not let an "expert" take your choices away from you. A 100-year-old man once said, "If I knew I was going to live this long, I would've taken better care of myself!"

12

ROOT-CANALS!

Root-Canals (Endodontics)

A root-canal!-An image that strikes terror in most people, ranking as the worst and most painful of all dental treatments. And well it should be a frightening prospect, but not just for the possible pain involved. The costs of a root-canal—both in monetary terms and to the overall health of the body—can be considerable.

As a potential root-canal patient, you cannot foresee the consequences of your treatment. Imagine that your tooth suddenly begins to hurt at 3:00 AM on a Sunday morning. The gums begin to swell. You have no pain medicine strong enough to help. Somehow you survive until Monday morning, when your dentist takes one look at you and says, "You need a root-canal."

Even though the thought of a root-canal is frightening, all you care about is stopping the pain. Often, these teeth are so tender that no treatment can be started. So the dentist usually gives you two prescriptions, one for a strong pain medicine to get you through the next few days and one for antibiotics to reduce the infection and keep it from spreading into the rest of your body.

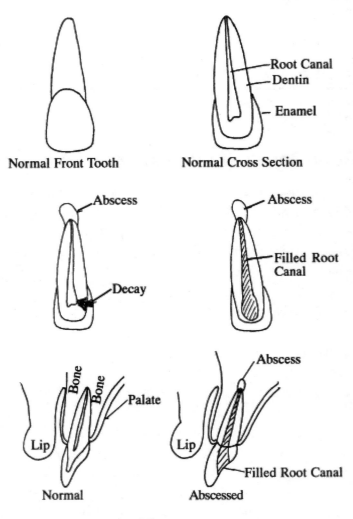

Abscesses

Figure 12.1

The pain in your mouth really comes from your body sending a large number of white blood cells into the area to fight the infection, causing swelling and pressure. The antibiotic reduces the level of bacteria, which in turn reduces the swelling, which in turn reduces the pain. (Many patients call a dentist when they are in awful pain and have swelling, but once the crisis has passed, they think they are "healed" and skip their appointment. A short while later, they call the dentist again because the pain is back and it is worse.)

Normally, after three to five days on the antibiotics, you return to your dentist or see a specialist, called an "endodontist." (The word "endodontist" means "dentist who treats the inside of teeth." The technical term for a root-canal is "endodontic therapy," but most people just say "root-canal," because that is the part of the tooth where the treatment is done.) After numbing the tooth, a hole is then drilled in the top of the tooth, just as if a filling were being done. The hole is deepened until the pulp chamber, the top end of the root-canal, is reached. The dentist now has access to the whole length of the root-canal. Most back teeth have more than one root-canal, with many having four.

Next, a series of treatments is begun which clean and shape the root-canal which are flushed, treated with chemicals to kill bacteria, and eventually filled with one of a variety of materials. The most common material is called gutta percha, a rubbery substance that is 15 percent barium to make it show up on X-rays. Another popular treatment used by 20 percent of American dentists is called the Sargenti method, but it is denounced by the ADA because it contains formaldehyde compounds and lead. The current formulas are said to have removed the lead, but tens of millions of root-canal treatments using the old formulas are still in people's mouths.

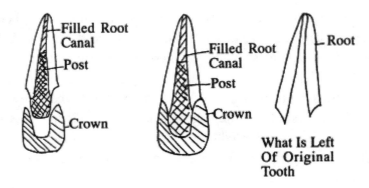

Root Canals

Figure 12.2

Once the root-canal treatment is completed, a patient is routinely told that a crown will be needed for strength because root-canal treated teeth become brittle and weak because of the inside having been drilled out to do the treatment. It is quite possible that there will be little of the original tooth left above the gum line and that which is left will be weak. In many cases, a post must be placed into the root-canal itself to hold the crown.

Many times the tooth may have been crowned before it dies. In fact, the ADA has reported that up to 20 percent of all teeth crowned will die. Consider this connection: Crowned teeth can die and then need root-canals; teeth that die and get root-canal treatments, need crowns. These two treatments are tightly interrelated. A tooth recommended for crowning can cost upwards of $600. Later, the tooth may die and cost another $500 for a root-canal. Or maybe a botched filling that cuts into the pulp chamber turns into a root-canal treatment followed by a crown. The economics behind these treatments is powerful, too powerful. However, the patient may not believe that the cost is the most important consideration, because both he and his dentist are trying to "save" the tooth by whatever means necessary. Since no one wants to lose his teeth, it all seems to work out—the patient saves his tooth and the dentists makes a living. Right? Well, consider a few additional problems.

A Tooth Is An Organ

A tooth is an organ, just as the heart or kidney or any bone in the body is an organ. An abscessed or gangrenous tooth is not only a dead tooth, it is a dead organ. The body does not like dead organs. The immune system does not recognize this now-dead tissue as part of itself and immediately sets out to eliminate or isolate it. The system must fight for as long as the tooth remains in the body and in many instances, it must fight against bacteria and toxins left after the tooth has been extracted.

Immune System Responses

The immune system tries to keep the infection in a small area in one or more of the following three ways: It forms a cyst or a granuloma, or it thickens the bone, which is called "condensing osteitis." If the infection is extensive, it will try to shunt the drainage to the outside of the body. The abscess can most commonly shunt on the outside of the tooth, but can also shunt into a sinus, on the roof of the mouth, or even through the skin. Once an abscess can drain, the pain-causing pressure drops and the acute (coming to a crisis quickly) infection subsides to a chronic infection (long-term, low-level pain).

339

As described above, the first step most dentists choose is to fight the infection with a prescription for antibiotics. It is a common misconception that antibiotics "heal." The truth is antibiotics only help the body overcome an infection; it is the body's immune system that must finish off the infection. Most, if not all, infections never completely go away. The levels of the bacteria just drop low enough so that they are no longer an acute threat.

Bacteria In The Body

Once a species of bacterium enters your body, you can never be 100 percent free of it. No pneumonia patient is ever free of the pneumonia bacterium. Likewise, no root-canal patient is ever free of the toxin-producing, anaerobic bacteria. (Anaerobic bacteria live where there is no oxygen and are always bad.) Small pockets of infection always remain and can become a threat again when the immune system becomes weak. In fact, the danger is that these chronic infections will actually cause the immune system to become weak.

During all the time a root-canaled tooth is kept in the mouth, the immune system has to deal with the chronic infection and the toxins, expending much energy to maintain normal health in the presence of this threat. Almost every healthy person has enough immune system reserves to keep one root-canal from becoming life threatening, but in some people this infection could be life threatening, for example people with damaged heart valves or HIV/AIDS. These people are especially at risk, particularly from an acute infection.

340

Anyone whose immune system is so depressed that they have a life-threatening illness would be wise to have their root-canal-treated teeth removed. But it is foolish to wait until your immune system is damaged before getting root-canals out, because doing it sooner may save you from such a crisis in the first place.

Chronic Drainage

It is common for the drainage from a tooth infection to have been present for so long that the body makes a drainage duct called a "fistula." A fistula is an external opening which looks like a small bump on the gums over the root, and which, when pressed, emits a little pus. To most people, this seems like a fine natural solution--no pain is felt; therefore no treatment is needed. Unfortunately, pain or not, your immune system is still at work and must continue to defend against this chronic infection. The tooth remains infected, whether it hurts or not. In fact, the less pain you feel the worse the infection may be because the body may not be containing the infection around the tooth but it is escaping into the body. Thus, the immune system has a much larger job to do in finding and destroying the escaped bacteria and toxins.

An abscessed tooth is a dead organ, whether it has had root-canal therapy or not. The body often tries to eliminate dead teeth, treated or not, by destroying the bone around the tooth. Given enough years, the immune system will destroy so much bone that the tooth will fall out. Every dentist has seen this happen and most common in teeth that have formed cysts or granulomas before the treatment was done.

It is also common for dentists to see people with as many as 10 root-canal-treated teeth. The burden to the immune system from this many root-canal-treated teeth can become a serious health challenge. Also, so much expensive dental treatment raises serious questions about whether the patient is being "over-treated" or whether these crowned teeth are dying after being treated because of how the dental work was done.

Devitalizating A Tooth

Some dentists think they can justify doing a root-canal even on a tooth that is still alive and healthy. It may be that he wants to reshape the tooth so much during a crowning procedure that the pulp chamber (nerve) will be exposed to the outside, which usually kills a tooth. The dentist may believe that getting the shape right is more important than leaving the tooth alive, so a "vital" root-canal will be done. In other words, to get a better-looking result, a living tooth will be killed. But patients would object to having a tooth killed, so the dentists use the term "devitalized." The ADA reports that root-canals done on "vital" teeth are more successful than root-canals done on abscessed teeth, the reason being obvious: No infection, cyst or granulomas are present to complicate the procedure.

The ADA makes doing root-canal therapy on living teeth sound like a great technique, but it misses the major point: A living tooth should be left alive. There is no valid reason to kill a tooth. If a technique requires a tooth to be devitalized (killed), then it is a bad technique.

The Effect of Dead Teeth on The Body

The root-canal-treated tooth is dead because the blood supply and nerve have been removed, leaving the patient with a "dead organ" in his body. What do physicians do with dead organs? They remove them! Dead kidney? Out! Dead foot? Cut it off! Physicians know that if a gangrenous organ is left in the body, the body could die from toxic shock.

So if dead organs need to be removed, why are dead teeth okay to leave in the body? One oral surgeon said it was okay because a tooth is a hard structure, but bones are hard structures, too, and physicians do not leave dead bones in the body. Physicians ignore dead teeth, leaving tooth decisions up to dentists, who are supposed to know what they are doing.

Defining Success

Unfortunately, initially the root-canal procedure appears to work. Millions are done each year with an often-estimated 95 percent success rate. But it depends on how "95 percent success" is defined. No pain, no complaints, no obvious swelling, no drainage? Usually, a dentist is satisfied if the patient is just free from pain, hoping that any other problem will go away in time. Freedom from pain but not from infection should not be considered a successful procedure.

Where The Bacteria Live

During a root-canal the main canal is filled and possibly some of the small side canals. But, the other, smaller canal-like structures in teeth, called dentinal tubules, are too tiny to be filled during treatment. Originally filled with cell extensions coming from the main cell bodies inside the once healthy root-canal, the tubules instead become home to bacteria. These tubules are wide enough for the bacteria to fit three abreast, and since there are millions of them, which when added together total several miles in length, there is room for enough bacteria to challenge the immune system. To a bacterium they are very large, virtual mansions. Inside these dentinal tubules bacteria remain safe because the white blood cells cannot penetrate from outside the tooth because the outer layer of the root, the cementum, blocks them. Tubules are perfect havens for the anaerobic (non-oxygen breathing) bacteria which are always a threat to the body.

These bacteria find enough to eat because fluids containing nutrients can enter the tubules from outside the tooth since the cementum can be penetrated by fluids, whose molecules are much smaller than the white blood cells. The waste products from these nasty germs include some toxic substances called thio-ethers. These toxins are poisonous and flow out of the tooth, just as the nutrients can enter. These foreign substances are picked up by the immune system and carried to the liver for detoxification. Unfortunately, the liver can be seriously damaged by them. The only way a dead tooth could remain in a body and not cause damage is if it is sterile and contains no deadly toxins, and there has never been a sterile, toxin-free dead tooth.

The reason root-canals seem relatively harmless is that no one traces the damage done to their body back to the infection within the tooth. The bacteria and toxins can spread to other organs through the blood vessels or the lymph system and tend to lodge in filtering organs like lymph nodes, the kidney and liver. In addition to these filtering organs bacteria in the body tend to go to weak areas, areas that are already inflamed. Here, they can cause further problems, none of which will be linked to the root-canal-treated tooth.

Physicians Are Dentally Blind

Dental procedures are not counted as a risk factor when a patient is checked for cirrhosis of the liver. If you were having liver problems, would you check with a dentist? Probably not. Physicians believe that the treatments dentists do have been thoroughly researched. Although they have been correctly taught that infections from the mouth can spread to any area of the body, they still do not routinely consider the possibility of dental origins for problems that are not adjacent to the mouth. This denial is changing. Physicians are beginning to find out how many of the chronic problems that have baffled them for decades, start in the mouth.

Damage Caused by Dental Infections

One of the well-known risks of dental treatment for some people is that of dying from an infection on the heart valves from bacteria released during the cleaning of teeth. Similarly, people with hip replacements must take antibiotics even for routine dental care because of the risk that bacteria entering the blood during dental treatment may lodge and multiply in areas of inflammation around the hip implant. This care is ironic because the inflammation that destroyed the joint initially may have been caused by dental problems resulting from mercury fillings and root-canals.

It comes back to which basic philosophy is right: "Save a tooth at any price" or "No tooth is worth damaging the immune system." That is the decision the patient must make. But in our era of autoimmune problems and chronic ill health, it seems foolish to aggravate our immune system by trying to maintain teeth that are dead. The time to act is before problems arise. "An ounce of prevention" is still better than a "pound of cure."

Detecting Problems In Advance

Unfortunately, a tooth can be seen but the immune system is hidden. A patient may think that a root-canal will only cause a little damage and getting one is no big deal. For a young and strong person, that may be true. A person may experience no major problems for years after a root-canal, but all the time the infection is festering. So what should you do if you have one or more root-canal-treated teeth? Is there a way to find if the root-canal is causing problems before they get out of hand?

Dentists are taught to do an annual X-ray of every root-canal-treated tooth. However, this type of X-ray, called a "periapical," meaning "around the end of the root," is rarely, if ever, done. Patients wanting to check on a root-canaled tooth need to ask their dentist to do the periapical X-ray. A dentist's trained eye can detect problems and help you see if there are any unhealthy changes. Specifically, look for:

1) A dark area around the root tip or along the side of the root, indicating the presence a cyst or granuloma;

2) A thickening of the bone, called "condensing osteitis" (bone infection or osteomyelitis). This thickening may appear on an X-ray as a wispy, white area surrounding the end of the root and is the body's attempt to contain the infection; and

3) An overfilled root-canal The filling in each root should end within one millimeter of the tip of the root; it should not stop farther up the canal than one millimeter or extend past the root tip.

If you see any of these three conditions, you are likely to have problems with your root-canal. These conditions, which are all indications of poor technique or gross infection, indicate that the tooth should be extracted, although the dentist may suggest other solutions, like redoing the root-canal or doing an apicoectomy, a procedure where the end of the root is removed.

What if you have more than one root-canal? This is not uncommon and may show that you have a general weakness in some of your body's basic systems that so weaken your teeth that they die. An unhealthy person tends to experience more damage from minor problems than a healthy person. A routine cavity in an unhealthy person may cause a tooth to die, whereas in a more healthy person the tooth would survive. On the other hand, several root-canals also may show that a dentist was too aggressive in his treatment. Many of the more elaborate dental procedures require that all teeth, even healthy ones, have root-canals done. These are obviously terrible treatment concepts and should be rejected, no matter how persuasive the dentist is.

Other Symptoms

Aside from the annual periapical X-ray, certain symptoms indicate problems. Do you feel any uncomfortable sensations coming from that tooth? Does the tooth "act up" now and then, particularly to hot or cold or from pressure when you chew? Does it have any drainage? Does it have any taste or smell? Do you notice a small bump on the gums over the root? Are you sick with some chronic (long-term) problem that no one can diagnosis? If any of these symptoms is present, the root-canaled tooth may need to be extracted.

Price of Procrastination

If you do not have the tooth extracted, you may be risking your total health for one tooth. Even without any symptoms, you must decide if you are willing to take the risk that more subtle damage is not going on in your body, damage that is not obvious to any dentist or physician until it becomes worse, and by then may be irreversible. The potential for root-canaled teeth to damage your health cannot be emphasized enough.

Extracting Root-Canal Teeth

If you do decide to have the tooth extracted, be aware of the following concerns. When these teeth are removed they can smell awful because they commonly have sacs of infection attached to the root or left in the socket. Thus, it is important that the socket be properly cleaned, or the bone may not fully heal (see "Extractions" and "Cavitations"). Also, root-canal-treated teeth can be the most difficult of all teeth to remove because they are so brittle. Roots commonly fracture, and the teeth routinely come out in little pieces, particularly the upper molars and bicuspids. By contrast, the surrounding bone may be spongy. On

348

the upper back teeth there may even be a hole directly into the maxillary sinus. After the extraction the sockets can bleed more than in non-infected extractions because of the extra blood supply needed by the immune system to fight the infection. All these problems can be minimized if your dentist uses the proper extraction techniques.

Deciding on a Root-Canal

If you do not have any root-canals and a dentist tells you one is necessary, what do you do? First, be sure you really have a problem. It is common for root-canals to be done on teeth that are merely "annoying." A dentist may feel that the tooth will die eventually and doing the procedure early is better than later. He may believe it will save you aggravation.

Many teeth that are annoying eventually self-heal, particularly if the problem is a heavy bite which occurs when one tooth hits another before the rest of the teeth come together, which commonly happens after a new filling because it is difficult to get the bite back to normal while the jaw is numb. The heavy bite causes inflammation within the tooth which makes the tooth cold sensitive, but can also happen as the teeth naturally shift. A heavy bite can be fixed simply by removing the offending high point. The low level of inflammation can usually be controlled with an over-the-counter painkiller. If an adjustment of the bite does not help and an over-the-counter pain pill does not control the pain, then a more serious situation may be developing. The need for a prescription painkiller is a sign the tooth may be dying.

349

Symptoms of an Abscess

Until definite symptoms of an abscess begin, no irreversible treatment should be done. Symptoms of a dying tooth are swelling, and sensitivity to hot and cold, pressure, and/or percussion (tapping). A dentist may test the tooth to see if it is still vital with an electrical device that can give a bit of a jolt, but this test may not be accurate. For example, in an upper molar, which has at least three roots, one may be dead or dying, but the other two could still be alive, thereby giving the tooth a positive reading, even though gangrene is present. An X-ray can also detect signs of abscess.

Making The Decision

The determination that the tooth is dying or dead brings the critical question: Should you have a root-canal done or just have the tooth extracted? It is easy for someone else to make a judgment, but you have to live with it. Absolutes are easiest: "Never have a root-canal done" or "Always have a root-canal to save the tooth." You are the one who must weigh the risks. Ask yourself, "Is doing a root-canal on this tooth worth damaging my immune system?"

For example, what if the tooth in question is a front tooth that was damaged in an accident and you are a healthy 20-year-old who still has all your other teeth? A quick root-canal, and the problem seems over. Having extraction and wearing a plastic tooth for the rest of your life seems like too much hassle. In many instances, it is less expensive to have the root-canal therapy than to have the tooth removed and replaced; this may be an example of a situation in which a person may wish to risk a root-canal. However, most situations will not be this clear-cut.

What if you are 40 and an upper second molar (the last tooth in the arch) abscesses? Although the tooth has not been crowned, it does have a large filling. If you do a root-canal and crown, you will spend over $1000. If you have the tooth extracted, it will cost much less and make only a small difference in chewing ability. This would be a definite "Get it out!" decision.

The Dentist's Attitude

Could you go ahead and get the root-canal and then later, when you have grown older, have it removed? The key is that you be informed of the consequences of the choices before you decide what is best for yourself. Your dentist may give you many apparently rational reasons for getting or keeping a root-canal. If you express doubt, you may be overwhelmed with all kinds of arguments. The dentist may tell you of success stories and satisfied patients. Many dentists get angry when a patient is reluctant to get a root-canal or have one removed and may even stop seeing you as a patient. Consider yourself lucky to get away from such a dentist.

To help you reach a decision, see the "Informed Consent" form shown in the Appendix I. Instead of the usual form a dentist asks you to sign for legal reasons, this one is for you to have the dentist fill out, so it is clear that if the treatment results in one of the bad effects described above, the dentist accepts some responsibility. Most dentists will not readily sign such a document, even if they expect you to sign one, but just using it to force the dentist to give straight answers about your treatment options will help you make better decisions.

Many dentists do not like to do root-canals, so they refer all such treatments to specialists. Other dentists do root-canals only on the easier front teeth and refer the back teeth to specialists. But because a specialist does the work does not mean there will not be problems. Many patients of both general dentists and specialists continue to suffer problems after their root-canal is completed. They are then prescribed several rounds of antibiotics, hoping they will end the problem but they usually do not work and problems eventually return.

Apicoectomy

The next treatment recommended is an "apicoectomy," which literally means "cutting off the end of the root," usually done by an endodontist or an oral surgeon. In most cases a mercury filling is placed in the end of the tooth to seal the canal. Now the patient has toxic mercury implanted within the jawbone, and if any scraps of the mercury material escape during treatment, they can spread into the bone. This escaped mercury can be impossible to remove even if the tooth is extracted.

An apicoectomy may end the patient's symptoms of pain and swelling, because a lot of acute infectious material is removed from the bone around the root end of the tooth. The patient stops complaining, which makes the dentist believe all is well, but the infection is not gone, but has, in fact, become chronic; the tooth can never be sterile. And do not forget the negative effects of the mercury in the bone.

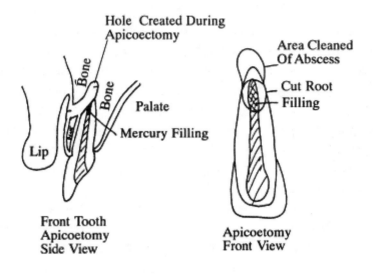

Apicoectomy

Figure 12.3

Why Dentists Love Root-Canal Therapy

Besides fulfilling the philosophy of saving teeth at any cost, dentists need to do root-canal therapy for another major reason. It has been said that physicians "bury" their mistakes. Well, dentists do root-canals on their mistakes! Root-canals are done on the 20 percent of crowned teeth that end up dying because of the damage done during the crowning procedure. If a dentist recommends a crown and the patient agrees, then six or twelve months later the tooth becomes sensitive, most dentists or patients do not put the two events together. They figure the tooth is dying and the next step is a root-canal. The crown the dentist did to "strengthen" the tooth is simply probably the cause of its death. If the dentist does connect the two treatments, it is easy to rationalize that since the tooth was in such a poor condition that it needed a crown, it would have died anyway. Translated, that means it is the patient's fault for not taking better care of his teeth.

Now to "save" the tooth after the damage done by crowning, the dentist must do a root-canal. If dentists did not have the root-canal procedure to bail them out, what would they do? They would have to say, "Gee, I'm sorry, Mr. Patient, that tooth I talked you into crowning has to be extracted!" Acceptance by the dentist of blame for the tooth dying will never happen. Besides, if dentists want to continue crowning teeth, which they are told constantly is the key to having a successful practice, they must have root-canal therapy to back them up. Of all the questionable treatments that dentists use, root-canal therapy may be the worse. The term "root-canal" should be changed to better explain just how bad the procedure is. The term "rot canal" is much more appropriate.

While root-canal therapy may be the worst procedure, it is also the backstop for most every other dental procedure. If the dentist does something wrong, root-canal therapy lets him cover the mistake. As a bonus, the dentist or the specialist picks up a nice extra fee. And to top it all, if the tooth does not already have a crown, one is always strongly recommended, because a root-canal tooth is prone to fracture. A dentist can turn a single mistake into several treatments that cost a thousand dollars of your money.

When you think about what 24 million root-canals a year generate in income for dentists, you can see why dentists will not want to give up the procedure. Would $8,000,000,000 (that is eight billion dollars) surprise you? Don't forget to add all the extra crowns needed to "protect" the treated teeth, another three billion dollars. Compare this total to how much all the Hollywood movies make in ticket sales in a year, about five billion dollars, and you can see just how powerful the economics are.

Pulpotomy For Baby Teeth

The endodontic procedure for infected baby teeth is called a "pulpotomy," which means "cutting off the pulp." And that is exactly what is done. An opening is made into the root-canal of the baby tooth, which is much wider than in adult teeth. After the tissue is removed, chemicals are used to clot the bleeding and a filling material is placed in the opening.

All the other problems associated with root-canals in adults apply to pulpotomies. The infection does not go away. Often, large abscesses form under these teeth which can drain at the side of the tooth. It is common to see a large swelling on the gums next to these teeth, which, if pushed, pus will come out.

Since the body sheds baby teeth naturally, the body may speed up the process, so the infected tooth falls out early. The whole purpose of keeping an infected baby tooth in the mouth is to hold the space open for the adult tooth growing beneath it. However, the possible complications may be a big price to pay. Pulpotomies are not recommended in this age of low immunity.

Crowning Baby Teeth

In many children dentists do the same as they would do to an adult; they crown or cap the problem tooth. Since the tooth will fall out in a year or two, a pre-formed crown is used, usually called a stainless steel crown. Remember, stainless steel is made with nickel and chromium, both highly carcinogenic (cancer-causing). If parents knew this, they would not allow this material to be used in their child's mouth.

Pedodontists, dentists who specialize in children's dentistry, love to do stainless steel crowns. It is quite common for them to do this treatment instead of fillings because it is faster and simpler than doing a filling and it makes lots of money. It may cost over $125 for one of these crowns, and a skilled dentist can put one on in minutes. The high fee and the short amount of time to do the procedure may make it the most lucrative procedure in dentistry. However, there is no justification for placing these dangerous metals in a child's mouth.

On top of the cancer risk nickel causes a hypersensitivity reaction in 10 percent of females and one percent of males. The chief symptom is depression. Would an artificially caused depression in a child between the ages of 4 and 11 affect his personality development? Certainly! The hazards of these treatments are not worth saving these teeth for a couple of years. The best answer is still prevention.

Avoiding Problems

Since no good options are available to prevent the crowding of permanent teeth when baby teeth have to be removed because of an abscess, prevention is the only solution. Instead of seeking ways of correcting damage caused by feeding junk food to our children, we should stop feeding them junk food. It is that simple.

Dentists commonly hear mothers telling them how their children insist on drinking too many sodas and eating too many sweets, but when they ask these mothers, "Who buys the sugary foods?" the answer is usually silence. They may get the message but the pressure from the advertisers and their children is relentless. It takes firm resolve to improve the family's eating habits because of resistance both from the children and the husbands. But children will eat what their parents give them, particularly if it is what the parents eat themselves.

Remember, the damage found in the mouths of our children is a direct result of choices that we as parents have made. The decay in a tooth is an outward symptom of deeper metabolic problems which can lead to unhealthy bodies and chronic, degenerative diseases, such as diabetes. Fixing the tooth and not addressing what is really causing the problem is, at best, shortsighted.

The Future of Root-Canal Therapy

Dentists do not want to give up doing root-canals. Root-canal treatment allows dentists to do many other money-making procedures, procedures that are unfortunately life threatening to teeth but are necessary to the economic viability of the modern dental practice. Many dentists hope that new root-canal treatments may actually sterilize teeth, which will allow the current dental procedures to continue unchanged. (However, even perfect sterilization will still not answer the problem of toxins.) The use of new chemicals and even lasers is said to be "promising," but the burden of proof is on the advocates of these new procedures and is mostly wishful thinking. The reality will remain the same. Prevention is the true answer. No treatment will ever be able to remove the toxins and bacteria from the dentinal tubules.

Recommendation: Never have root-canal therapy done to any tooth, adult or baby. If you have had root-canals done, you should plan to have them removed, but only by someone who follows the procedures outlined under the section on "Extractions." Any other course of action may present unacceptable risks to your long-term health.

13

PULLING TEETH CAN CAUSE PROBLEMS

Extractions

There are worse things than losing a tooth.
Anonymous

To extract means "to take something out," in this case, a tooth from the mouth. People seldom call a dental office and say they need an "extraction." Usually it is, "Can I get a tooth pulled?" They may say "jerked out" or even "yanked." The last two terms give dentists cold chills. These terms rank at the top of popular dental terms that dentists hate. (Other terms dentists hate are pyorrhea, plate, tooth mechanic and the excuse, "I forgot my checkbook!")

There is more to removing teeth than people think. First, teeth are not pulled, but are elevated or lifted out using leverage. Most teeth are attached to the bone so strongly that a dentist could not pull it out, no matter how strong he was. The usual procedure is to loosen the tooth by rocking it back and forth or side to side in the socket.

Once the tooth is loose, it is grasped by specially designed forceps ($100 pliers) and tipped back and forth until it is loose enough to come out.

359

How Teeth Are Attached

Teeth are not directly attached to the bone. There are three layers of tissue between the tooth and the bone: The periosteum, a tough thin layer that surrounds every bone; the cementum, a thin layer that covers the dentin of the root; and the peridontal (meaning "around the tooth") ligaments which are tiny, but numerous, fibrous connectors between the cementum and the periosteum. (See Fig. 1.2 on page 13.) These ligaments act as shock absorbers to the teeth. They have nerve sensors that allows us to tell how hard food is so we know how much pressure to use when we chew. If you were eating mashed potatoes and bit into a BB, these are the nerves that would react.

The periodontal ligaments are also the reason teeth can be moved with orthodontics. When teeth are moved, tension on one side stretches the fibers, which stimulates bone growth and pressure on the other side causing the bone to reabsorb. Slowly, the tooth can be moved through the bone.

Individually, these tiny ligaments are weak, but there are millions of them. To remove a tooth, the dentist uses leverage to break enough fibers that the tooth can be removed. This procedure is easier to do on one-rooted teeth, like the eight front teeth, than it is on the two-rooted bicuspids or the multi-rooted molars. Each tooth is unique and has a specific technique for removal. Many specialized elevators and forceps are available to allow removal of the teeth with minimum damage to the surrounding bone. But just getting the tooth out is not enough. The socket must be properly cleaned, so complete healing can occur.

Tissue Remnants

Those three layers mentioned earlier lose their purpose, once the tooth is removed. Unfortunately, the layers do not all come out with the tooth. If we viewed the surface of the bone after an extraction with a microscope, we may see that the periosteum still covers the bone and also see torn pieces of the ligaments and cementum; if left, these tissues form a barrier to complete healing.

The new blood vessels that should form after an extraction are stopped by the remnants of the tough periosteum. Without these new blood vessels new bone cannot form. Therefore, it is important that the dentist clean the surface of the bone so there are none of these tissues left to interfere with healing. Most dentists do not even attempt to remove this tissue. Once the tooth is out, they put a piece of gauze in and say, "Bite."

Extraction Technique

The most important way to have complete healing is proper extraction technique, which helps in the immediate postoperative symptoms and the long-term healing of the bone. If the bone cannot heal properly, a cavitation may form (See "Cavitations.").

Dentists were not taught these concepts in dental schools 30 years ago and it probably has not improved. Learning to do extractions is stressful and just getting the tooth out seems like the job is done. Most dentists believe that once the tooth is out, all they need to do is put in a folded piece of gauze and tell the patient to bite down, plus instructions to put ice or cold compresses on it.

It is important that once a tooth is extracted the socket is cleaned of all tissues except the healthy bone. This task requires both cleaning with hand instruments and both high speed and slow-speed drills. All the while, the area must be flushed with antiseptic solutions or sterile water. Any tissue left may interfere with complete healing. Dentists do not like to do this stressful cleaning, as they are afraid of damaging other structures, such as a nerve, blood vessel, or sinus. None of these structures should be damaged, if the dentist is careful and knows his anatomy. Another reason dentists do not like to clean the socket, as described, is that they or their staff must sterilize clean all the extra instruments.

Once the socket is clean, a clot-inducing form of gelatin (Gelfoam) can be placed, which oral surgeons use in difficult surgeries. If it helps then why not use it for all surgeries? It is expensive, about two dollars per piece, but aren't you worth it? Following the placing of the Gelfoam the gums should be stitched as tight as possible over the socket. This procedure, too, is counter to dental training but it seems reasonable that the smaller the opening the better and faster the healing. This procedure also costs time and money, as suture setups are expensive. Doing all the above is a lot of extra work compared to putting a piece of gauze and saying, "Bite on this," but it is worth it to achieve faster and easier healing.

Here is one that shocks all dentists, physicians and nurses: Instruct the patient to use hot compresses, not cold. When this concept is brought up the usual response is "sputtering." The idea is so ingrained to use cold that it seems heresy to suggest that is the wrong thing to do, but it is. Cooling the site reduces the number of white blood cells available to attack bacteria that have invaded the socket and bone. Even in the best technique, millions of the little critters get in. Cooling the area allows them a head start that may cause much trouble. More sputtering. "But you'll have bleeding problems," they finally challenge. Excess bleeding does not seem to occur and might even make the platelets work better, creating a more solid clot.

In a recent study medical surgical patients were cooled, thinking that it would be easier on them. They were cooled only a few degrees. The result was they had three times more post-op infections. Heat heals. All those sports figures getting iced down (and it is very painful) may be doing the opposite of what is needed for real healing.

If that suggestion causes sputtering, try this: Take ibuprofen or aspirin pre-op. "You can't do that. It causes bleeding," they cry in unison. That's their theory but it does not seem to work that way in our office. The way these drugs work is they need to be present before the pain messages are sent to the brain. If you wait until the messages of pain are sent to the brain, it takes much longer for them to be effective.

If there is any post-op bleeding that requires more than one gauze pad, the homeopathic (sputter, sputter) ferrum phos is given. The bleeding seems to come under control in seconds, inexplainable in traditional terms, but it works like a charm.

While mentioning homeopathics, some help patients heal quickly. Arnica is the chief one that has been used for a century with great success. Ruta and hypericum are also given with the arnica after the extraction and are sent home with the patients to be used every half-hour for about eight hours.

It is common for patients not to need any further pain relief, even after an hour-long surgical procedure. The occurrences of post-op infections are almost nonexistent. So, any dentist sputtering, please keep an open mind and try these ideas. You may be pleasantly surprised. If you are the patient, it will be difficult to change the dentist's technique. You can do some of it yourself. It is common for alternative-oriented patients to know what they want and avoid most of the dentist's instructions.

The techniques described above change as treatments evolve. In six months from this writing, techniques might differ in significant ways. To find changes, check our website (**dentistry-toothtruth.com**).

Cavitations

If tissue is left in the socket, the bone will tend to heal over the top, leaving a hole in the bone. This hole can persist for the rest of a patient's life, a chronic infection called a "alveolar cavitational osteopathosis." This term means that there is an infected (patho) cavity in the bone (osteo) that held the tooth (alveolus). Other terms used are "cavitation" or NICO (Neural Inducing Cavitational Osteopatosis) or even osteomyelitis.

New Research

These bone infections are only now being seriously researched. The first research papers came out in the mid-1980's and are mostly a dentist-caused problem which most dentists do not know they are causing. Cavitations are quite common and visible on X-rays, appearing as an empty tooth socket, even though it might have been years or decades since the tooth was removed. When dentists see them on an X-ray, they do not know what they are looking at so pass them over as "normal." Dentists were told that these were "healed extraction sites" when they were really "unhealed extraction sites," so common that most extraction sites have one, particularly wisdom-tooth sites. These chronic infections can cause chronic health problems from mild to severe.

If these infections are fairly easy to prevent by proper socket cleaning, then why is this cleaning not being done? Many, if not most dentists, have never heard about cavitations and their cause. Once the problem is taught in dental schools, it will slowly become part of the standard extraction technique. This process will take years once it begins, and it will be even longer before dentists routinely clean up the cavitations already formed. Probably less than a thousand dentists are currently willing to treat them.

Even if there is an obvious cavitation on an X-ray, very few of even those thousand dentists will suggest treating it because it is such a new procedure. Dentists are wary of doing anything different than their colleagues. In the next decade the cleaning and healing of these cavitations will grow in importance and be commonly done, at least for oral surgeons. While cleaning the cavitations may produce complete healing, it may also produce only partial healing. That means a cavitation may need to be redone until it completely heals.

The tooth sites the most likely to form cavitations are the wisdom teeth and any extraction that turns into a "dry socket." These locations have damaged bone that are routinely slow to heal.

Treatment

How do you decide to have a cavitation done if one is found? Unless you happen to be going to one of those 1000 dentists and actively ask that any cavitation be treated, you will probably have little success in getting them done. Unfortunately, for now there are few options.

Case History: A patient in her late forties had a "knot" or lump under the skin along the side of her lower jaw that had been there for years. X-rays of the teeth nearby did not show anything. When the area was checked surgically, a cavitation was found where a wisdom tooth had been removed 30 years earlier. The cavitation was treated. The next day, the knot grew larger and turned black and blue, showing that bleeding at the wisdom tooth site had flowed through the tissues to the "knot." That means the "knot" was a concentration of infectious material from the cavitation. After the cavitation site healed fully, the "knot" disappeared.

If the infection from a cavitation can flow to a spot in the cheek, it can go elsewhere, maybe to the lymph nodes or directly to the blood and can definitely be picked up by the white blood cells. This woman had had a chronic infection for on 30 years! How much work had the immune system had to do to control it during all those years? All that work could have been prevented by a few extra minutes of cleaning the tissue after the extraction. Complete healing is well worth the extra effort.

Unfortunately, many dentists are reluctant to clean sockets because it requires using many extra instruments, greatly increasing the amount of clean up required and making more things to be sterilized. Also, many dentists are no longer willing to do any surgical procedures. More dentists may stop doing any surgery because it vastly simplifies sterilization. Dentists also believe this procedure reduces the possibilities of their being contaminated with a patient's blood which may contain hepatitis or HIV. Since it is illegal to refuse to treat an HIV/AIDS patient, even if you could tell who they are in the first place, these dentists will not do any extractions, let alone more complex surgical procedures, a sound means by which a dentist protects himself in our over-regulated country.

Drysocket

The term "dry socket" is one that people seem to remember. The dental term is "septic socket," which means infected socket. Dry socket happens when the body is unable to maintain a blood clot in the socket of an extracted tooth, due to a low ionic calcium concentration. Once the clot is lost, an opportunistic bacterial infection can occur.

If you have an injury on your skin, it will bleed until a blood clot forms. The blood clot then hardens, which we call a scab. The same process happens when a tooth is extracted. Unlike the skin, the mouth is full of saliva, so the clot never fully hardens.

If bacteria can establish an infection between the clot and the bone, the clot may be lost, which leaves the socket empty or "dry." This result is bad, because bone exposed cannot heal because it cannot form a new clot. The bone is also living tissue so it is sensitive (hurts!).

Standard Treatment

The standard dental treatment is to prescribe antibiotics and put a sedative, engenol, the major ingredient in oil of cloves, in the socket to stop the pain. This sedative stops the symptoms. But what it really does is to help insure that a cavitation will form.

What is needed is for a new clot to be formed after the dead bone is removed. This procedure is a lot more trouble than giving a prescription and using some clove oil. But establishing a good blood clot will save having to treat a cavitation later or worse, leaving an unhealed infection in the bone for the rest of a patient's life.

Risk Factors

The risk factors for getting a dry socket are: Having an infection to begin with, such as an abscessed tooth; having extensive oral surgery done; that the tooth removed had had a root-canal treatment, meaning it was already infected; having poor healing ability, as in being run down or systemic illness, such as diabetes; being a smoker; and being a lower extraction versus an upper one. Many people have several of these risk factors. From experience, it seems that smokers are the worse risk group.

Ways to reduce the risks of a dry socket are: Pre-extraction antibiotics; taking specific vitamins that aid in healing, such as vitamins C and A; not smoking; proper cleaning of the socket, especially if it was a root canal-treated tooth; using Gelfoam, a form of gelatin that helps clots form; and closing the socket by suturing (stitches) to hold the clot in and keep mouth fluids out. If you need to have any extractions done, get yourself in as healthy condition as possible before it is done. Prevention is better than treatment!

Wisdom Teeth

The third molars are commonly called "wisdom teeth," the molars that come in between ages 16 and 21.

In America wisdom teeth are usually stopped from coming in because of lack of space; when this happens, it is called

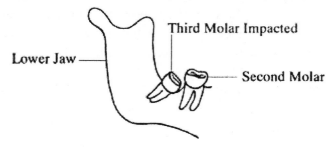

Impacted Wisdom Tooth

Figure 13.1

an "impaction," as in "my wisdom teeth are impacted." This blocking the tooth from erupting into a normal position is mostly due to the jawbone being too short to hold all the teeth in proper position. Impaction of these teeth often causes many problems, including damaged gum tissue and infection. The impaction of teeth is reason enough to have them removed. But many people feel that if the tooth is not bothering them, they should not bother it. Many would rather not even know that the teeth are impacted, the "ignorance is bliss" approach to problems.

Infections of The Wisdom Teeth

When an infection occurs, it is called "pericornitis;" meaning around (peri-) the crown (corn-) there is an infection (-itis). This infection can be very painful and serious and strikes young adults, usually at the most trying of times. It is common for these infections to occur during finals week at college. Students are cramming, not eating right and not sleeping much. The stress builds, the immune system weakens. A small chronic infection that may not have even been noticed becomes a full-blown, acute infection. The term "blows up" is appropriate; it happens fast, with pain and swelling. In 24 hours the whole side of the face may be so swollen that the eye cannot open. The mouth may only open a quarter inch.

If the student is lucky, he can get a prescription for antibiotics and pain pills. At best, it takes a week to get under control. A student may mess up a couple of grades. A worker may be fired for missing work. AND THE TEETH STILL HAVE TO BE EXTRACTED!

Please do not do this to yourself. Get the teeth out before they can cause trouble, especially before going to college or starting a full-time job. It is wise to get it done while still covered by parents' insurance. Many college students wait until they graduate, just before their insurance stops. It is better not to wait that long. The added risk of having an infection before the teeth are removed, even with the use of antibiotics, makes for slow healing and increases the risks of a "dry socket."

Why Do We Have Wisdom Teeth?

This is a question many patients ask. We have wisdom teeth for the same reason we have front teeth. Have you ever asked, "Why do we have front teeth?" Probably not, because they do not cause problems. So the question should be, "Why do wisdom teeth cause problems?" Are they left over from caveman days when our mouths were bigger and will they eventually disappear from human beings? These are possibilities, but it is much more probable that the problem is caused by us. The truth may be found by looking at people in other countries, countries with a more natural diet than ours.

When Dr. Weston Price toured the world in the 1930's, he found that it was the influence of Western diet that had the most to do with the improper growth of the body, including the jaws which hold the teeth. When the jaws do not develop to their full size, they are too short to hold all 32 teeth. The last ones in are the wisdom teeth, and there is no room left. This crowding is also seen with the eye-teeth (canine or cuspid) which may come in like tusks in people with small arches. We do not wonder if we will be losing our eye-teeth (canine or cuspid) through evolution. If you consider the full meaning of this information, you will understand that this same lack of space caused by our diet is the reason that millions of American teenagers continue to need braces year after year.

Have you ever wondered how the billions of poor people around the world get along without an orthodontist to handle all their crooked teeth? For the most part they don't need them because their teeth are not crooked. Having orthodontists to fix our kids is not a luxury Americans can afford because we are a rich country, but because our diet causes the crowded teeth. And the more generations that are on the Western diet, the worse the problem becomes. The solution has been known for generations but the only response by the dental schools is to produce more orthodontists. (See "Braces.")

Treatments Needed

You may already be past the cause and you want solutions. Is there any other way but extracting the wisdom teeth? In the vast majority of people the only answer is to get them out and go on with your life. Moaning about it does not help and probably does not get you much sympathy because we all have to face the same problem.

Removal of wisdom teeth between ages 17 and 20 will have little impact on your life; look at it as preventive maintenance. The bottom line is, get them out before they cause trouble.

What about the rest of us who are a bit wimpy about it? Can we not just wait until they bother us; really hoping that day never comes? This is America and you can do anything you want, but what will probably happen is when you can least afford to have problems, BOOM! One will blow up with an infection.

Even if these teeth manage to come in, they are still a problem. It is common to see such patients in their 50's and 60's with damage caused by wisdom teeth. At best, they are crowded, which makes them difficult to clean, easy to decay, difficult to fill, and damaging to the back of the second molar. No matter how you look at it, 95 percent or more of us should get them out and get on with our lives.

Methods of Extraction

Okay, you are convinced to get your wisdom teeth out. What is the best way to do it so there is a minimum of inconvenience and, especially, NO PAIN? Tall order, but it can be much less trouble than you think. The position of the wisdom teeth is important; some will be almost in, close to a normal position, while others can be so buried that they are upside down. Most will be coming in at an angle where they catch on the second molar and cannot quite straighten up. (See Fig. 13.1, page 369.) The position will determine who should remove them.

Each dentist who does extractions will have a level of difficulty they feel is beyond their skill and will refer those patients to an oral surgeon. Patients with special health problems, which could make a routine extraction life threatening, should also be referred. Many dentists have stopped doing any extractions and will refer all patients. Once it is determined who will do the surgery, there are two main ways to have them removed.

The first way is to have one side done at a time, usually done by a general dentist. While this method requires two healing periods, neither will be as difficult as having all four teeth done at once and also gives the patient a side to chew on during healing. Most patients do quite well doing two at a time. It may be less expensive to have a general dentist do the surgery. Since you already know your dentist, you may be more comfortable with him doing the work, rather than going to a specialist.

The second way is to have all four teeth done at one time. (There are four wisdom teeth, one in each corner.) If you are afraid to go through surgery twice, then this is your best way. While your courage is high, the oral surgeon will get all four teeth. Some general dentists will do all four at once, too.

Oral surgeons commonly use Valium IV sedation. Occasionally, a general anesthetic is required and you will have to go to the hospital, usually as an outpatient. After a couple of days to a week, you will be back to normal.

Whether a general dentist nor a specialist does the extractions, they need to be done as described in the section

373

"Extractions." It is important that the sockets are properly cleaned as wisdom teeth are on the heart meridian. An infection left in the bone may have serious health effects.

If neither the general dentist nor the specialist will follow the technique described, you should consider waiting until you find someone who does know the technique. If a cavitation develops after the extraction, which is common, another surgical procedure must be done later to correct the cavitation. It is better to just have the job done right the first time.

Recommendations

Try to have your wisdom teeth removed CORRECTLY, as soon as they are ready. A panoramic X-ray taken at age 16 will show how fast they are maturing. The optimum time to have them removed is after they have come through the bone but before they cut through the gums. This removal allows full access to properly clean the sockets to prevent cavitations and gives enough tissue to suture the opening for quick healing. To avoid most problems, they should be removed before a person is 20.

If you are over 40, and have luckily avoided problems, it may be best to do nothing. But it is not a good idea to hope you will be one of these people. A problem may still occur when you are 70 and be life threatening. If you get them out when you are young, you will be better off for the rest of your life.

14

REPLACING MISSING TEETH

Removable Partial Dentures

When one or more teeth are missing, they can be replaced with removable partial dentures, commonly referred to as "partials." These dentures are composed of the replacement teeth and the base, which has two functions, holding the teeth and fitting within the mouth so the partial stays in place. The replacement teeth are made of either plastic or porcelain. The base of the partial may be made out of plastic, which is found in almost every partial and/or various metals including chromium, nickel, and cobalt, plus many trace metals.

The shape of partials varies greatly, depending on the number of teeth being replaced, the type of materials, the shape of the mouth and the position of the remaining teeth. Every partial is custom-made to fit one person and range from simple to complex, with varying ways to attach them to the remaining teeth.

"Flippers"

Simple partials are used for people who are missing one or two teeth, commonly the upper front teeth. These simple plastic partials are called "flippers," because they can be flipped out with the tongue. Most people wear their "flippers" for years with no trouble, including some, which fit poorly, while still others can barely tolerate even well designed, attractive partials. The patient's attitude plays an important part in the success of wearing any partial denture. Patients with partials need to be routinely checked by a dentist to catch new problems early, but seem to be the least inclined to do so.

Many plastic partials have wire arms or "clasps" which help to hold them in place. These wire clasps contain nickel, a highly carcinogenic metal. Having any nickel in your mouth should be avoided.

Metal Partials

The most common partial is a metal one made of a chromium-cobalt alloy. This material makes a long-lasting and functional type of partial. It is not uncommon for these partials to last 20 years, although the natural changes in the teeth and gums over 10 years means these partials can cause some unwanted wear on the teeth.

Unfortunately, chromium-cobalt partials present a few major problems. First, the metals from which these partials are made are nickel, chromium and cobalt, all carcinogens. While little metal ever leaves the partial, some of it may be absorbed, and it does not take much of these toxic metals to create a toxic level in the body. Wearing these metals in the mouth for 20 years may well be an unreasonable risk that people should only take if they are informed before such a partial is made. Nevertheless, it is a risk millions of people are unaware they are taking. Deciding which type of partial is a good example of when an "Informed Consent" form should be used. (See Appendix I.)

Second, when wearing partials, any visible metal is unattractive. Most areas that show can be made with pink plastic gums and white plastic teeth, but the clasps are usually difficulty to hide. The best teeth to use are plastic ones. Porcelain teeth are not recommended because they can cause considerable damage by excessive wearing of the remaining natural teeth and also tend to chip, turn black where they fit into the plastic, and occasionally fall out.

Finally, the metal in a partial denture can create strong electric currents, which may be stronger than those created by fillings, because the partials contain more metal spread over a larger area than either fillings or crowns. Partials may actually connect many metal fillings and crowns as if they were wired together. In addition, metal partials electrically connect the right and left sides of the body, a situation that runs counter to the natural way the nerves of the body are arranged. The nerve paths in our bodies are specific in that they go to one side or the other and do not cross the mid-line of the body. Although we lack full knowledge of the effects of electric currents generated by dental metals, it is thought by many health practitioners that the amount of electricity metal partials generate should be enough to make using them a bad idea.

Flexite Partials

Until recently patients had no other choice than to use a metal partial, but now a new type of flexible plastic called Flexite is available. Flexite partials are made by dental labs under a franchise arrangement with the manufacturer. If a dentist's regular dental lab does not have the franchise, his lab can send the work to a second lab that does. In other words, Flexite partials are available to every dentist. While these partials will not last as long as the metal partials, they are a good compromise between function and biocompatibility, and the cost is comparable to the metal partials.

Flexite partials can be made with clear plastic except where gum areas are visible, which can be overlaid with a bit of pink plastic. Since this pink color is due to a metal coloring agent, as little as possible should be used.

It is also possible to make a unilateral partial, one that replaces one or two back teeth. (See Figure 11.7, page 323.) These small partials seem to work quite well as an alternative to cemented bridges. Most importantly, they eliminate the need for the dentist to cut down teeth for crowns as is necessary for a cemented bridge.

Another non-metal partial material is called Valplast, which has been available for decades. This material works well but has two drawbacks: It is hard to polish and Valplast cannot be easily relined. It is a good alternative to Flexlite if a dentist has a dental lab that can make it and he can get a good polish after adjustments.

Complete Denture Materials

A complete denture, made when all the teeth are missing, is also called dentures, false teeth, or plates. Most dentists prefer the term "dentures" and hate the term "plates," which is an old term but still commonly used by the general public. Dentures are a symbol of the ultimate failure of dentistry because all the teeth have been lost for one reason or another (usually diet-related gum problems). Fortunately, most people who wear complete dentures do so successfully, although if were not possible to make dentures, perhaps people would be more concerned about the causes of dental problems.

Patients have one main choice for the material to use for the denture base (the gum part of the denture)--acrylic (methyl methacrylate); this will be the right choice for the vast majority of people. Some special lab processes do use other materials, but unless you are allergic to acrylic, do not use anything else.

If you are a highly allergic person, you may wish to have a compatibility test done before having the denture made. It is even possible to test yourself by having a flat disc of denture acrylic made (about the size of a quarter) and taping it to your skin for a few days. If you are allergic, the skin under the disc will itch and turn red. If the skin begins to itch, stop the test if it does not do either, then acrylic should be an acceptable material for your dentures.

Coloring Agents

Usually, denture bases are made of one of many pink-colored acrylics. The pink color is created by metal coloring agents, usually cadmium but occasionally mercury, just as in partials. As with other dental materials containing mercury, mercury-containing acrylics should never be used. A major effect of cadmium is raising of blood pressure. While it is not known if the cadmium in dentures contributes to high blood pressure, it is prudent to minimize exposure and any metal used to color the denture can leach out over time. While the amount may be small, it does not take much to affect some people, and no one knows who is susceptible.

You can greatly minimize the amount of pink acrylic used by requesting that areas of the denture that cannot be seen be made of clear acrylic. The labs do not usually charge extra to have the denture made with a clear palate.

A new type of dental acrylic has been introduced that is called cadmium-free. The existence of such a product shows that there is concern by some dentists and manufacturers with the use of cadmium. The cadmium has been replaced by iron, manganese and cobalt oxides. Cobalt is a carcinogen.

It is possible that many dentists do not know that dentures are colored by metals. Pink acrylic is accepted without question. (Dentists accept too many aspects of their profession without question!) Ask your dentist to show you the Material Safety and Data Sheet (MSDS) on the acrylic he wants to use. Dentists are required by federal law to have the MSDS on all products they use in their offices. Ask for an explanation of the materials. Your dentist may learn more about them than you!

15

BRACES (ORTHODONTICS)

Dangers of Braces (Orthodontics)

Orthodontics means "to straighten teeth," which is done by using braces. The use of braces has become commonplace in America, not only because we are so rich that we can afford to have them, but because we eat and chew so poorly that we need them. Once the damage is done, braces may be the only way to correct the problem. We should however, try to improve our diets so children of the next generation can return to the natural, full, rounded arches where there is room for all our teeth. Presently, no one is even discussing the role of proper nutrition to prevent the deformations of the arches that require braces to (partially) correct. This information has been available for over 60 years, since Dr. Weston Price published his landmark book, *Nutrition and Physical Degeneration.*

If the cause of the problem is known, then why has the need for orthodontics gotten more widespread? As with most problems, follow the money. Money is made in supplying us with processed, inferior foods which lead to the need for braces. Then there is the money to be made in correcting the problem once it occurs. The only people interested in prevention are the ones paying, not those who reap the profits from causing and correcting problems. Unfortunately, the ones who pay mistakenly trust the professionals to help them correct problems instead of being aware of the causes themselves.

The truth is that most medical problems are self-induced. Individually, we have the ability to determine our future health and until we accept the responsibility, we are vulnerable to those who will shortchange our health for monetary gain.

The Reality of Wearing Braces

Braces have become a status symbol among teenagers, even a rite of passage. The reality of braces is two years of appointments, a mouth full of irritating (and toxic) metals, some pain, a lot of discomfort, and thousands of dollars. Doesn't all of this seem like something to avoid if possible? While it will take a major effort to revamp our eating habits to avoid needing orthodontics, such a change would have other blessings, namely, preventing and curing other health problems. Until that day comes, we are stuck with having crowded teeth or wearing braces because individually, we need to do what we can to correct the dental problems that already exist, which means braces for many kids.

While that may be the true of the current generation, we need to work on improving our eating habits, so the next generation may avoid these problems. Unfortunately, most grandparents tend to go the other way and give more "junk food" treats than they did as parents. While they do it out of love for their grandchildren, the real legacy of such doting is the degradation of the children's health.

It is important that people wearing braces maintain a consistent high level of oral cleanliness. It is common to see damage and decay on the teeth in the area between the brackets and the gums and to see long-term gum problems caused by poor cleaning habits. A low-sugar diet and better oral hygiene must be maintained. Soft drinks are a major problem. Damage can happen in just a few months, with teenage boys seemingly the most susceptible. Parents must make their concerns known to the orthodontists so that they are informed if their child is not doing a thorough job taking care of their braces.

Dental Materials Used In Braces

There are enough problems with braces without any other complications, but the dental materials used are a major cause for concern. The major toxic problem with braces is that the metals used in them can contain nickel and chromium, with nickel being the most carcinogenic metal. The possibility of nickel and chromium causing cancer is well known. Why nickel is allowed to be used in dentistry is a matter of convenience and cost. Nickel is used for crowns because it is the cheapest metal and in braces, has the best properties necessary to do the job. The cancer connection is simply an unfortunate possibility that seems to be ignored. If most parents knew of this potential problem, they would have grave concerns about its use in their children. We should be shown definitive studies showing that there is no possibility of developing cancer from using these metals before they are approved for continued use.

Nickel Hypersensitivity

What may be more common and immediate is a hypersensitive reaction to nickel, which happens in ten percent of girls and one percent of boys, a high percentage for a side effect.

The main symptom is depression, which may manifest in dropping grades, and personality changes like becoming sullen and withdrawn. Urinary tract problems may also occur because of the growth of nickel-dependent bacteria.

Parents may ignore these symptoms because they are difficult to distinguish from other common teenage behaviors and attitudes. But, since suicide is another potential problem associated with depression, parents must pay attention to any behavioral changes. Therefore, do not dismiss any behavior change in your child after getting braces because it may well be a result of a hypersensitivity to nickel. If you are an adult who has braces, you must monitor yourself.

Although the length of time the carcinogenic nickel in the braces is present in the mouth is only a few years, it is common for retainers with nickel wires to be used for years after the braces have been removed. It is also common for a nickel wire to be bonded to the backs of the lower teeth and left there indefinitely, usually until the patient reaches his twenties and gets tired of it. The long-term use of these nickel-containing wires could pose a serious exposure to toxic metals of which wearers of these devices should be aware.

As with all dental procedures, the reality is different than the image. It is always better to avoid the need for dental treatment than to worry about the possible damage from the materials used. Since there are no cures in dentistry, patchwork repairs for rotted teeth, surgery for only gum disease, braces for crowded teeth, and extraction when all else fails, prevention is always the best answer.

16

WHAT'S THE TRUTH ABOUT FLUORIDATION?

Fluoride causes more human cancer death, and causes it faster, than any other chemical.

Dean Burke, former Chief Chemist,
National Cancer Institute

Fluoridated Water

Fluoridation, still a controversial subject to many people, will become more controversial in the years ahead. However, it is not controversial to most American dentists who accept the ADA's pro-fluoride position as readily as they accept the ADA's pro-mercury position. Perhaps because of this wide acceptance influenced by the ADA, many Americans do not know that most European countries, which fluoridated their water at one time, have stopped doing it. The only major countries left with pro-fluoridation positions are the U.S., Canada, and Great Britain.

The question that needs to be asked is, "Why would fluoridation of public water be stopped if it is such a helpful and safe public health service?" The answer is that fluoridated water is not considered safe in these other countries. Statistics do not now, nor have they ever, supported the use of fluoride; if they had, Americans' teeth would be in far better condition than they are.

Even if the use of fluoride were a good idea, putting it in the drinking water is a poor way to deliver it. Fluoride in public water is a prescription medicine being given to the whole population, a medicine no one knows for sure how much anyone is taking or whether it is even needed. And if fluoride is a systemic poison, which it is, then this is a terrible thing to do to people in the name of stopping a few cavities per person per lifetime.

But for now, let us make a few assumptions: water fluoridation is a good idea; fluoridation doesn't cause cancer, even though it does; fluoridation does not cause bone damage and increased hip fracturing, even though it does; fluoride is always added to the water correctly, which it is not; everyone drinks the right amount of fluoridated water for their needs, but not a drop more, even though none of us knows what our need is; no one gets a maximum dose of fluoride from other sources, which happens often; the fluoride added is the same kind found in naturally fluoridated waters, which it is not. Actually, let's just forget all these assumptions because there are too many variables to justify the use of fluoridated water as a delivery system for a prescription drug!

Even if your tap water is not fluoridated, it is difficult to avoid fluoridated water, because it is used in the making of most processed foods and drinks. Fluoride is all around us, so while you should try to avoid it, you will still eat or swallow some and maybe a lot. Because fluoride is actually so pervasive, you should try to avoid it whenever you can.

Fluoride Researcher Changes Mind

Canada's leading fluoride authority and former fluoride promoter has reversed his position. Dr. Hardy Limeback, D.D.S., Ph.D., head of the Department of Preventive Dentistry of the University of Toronto and president of the Canadian Association for Dental Research, announced he had unintentionally misled the public. " We were wrong," he said. The toxicology information has been available for 15 years but we "had to refuse to study it."

He states that Toronto, which has been fluoridated for 36 years, has a higher rate of decay than Vancouver, which has never had fluoride. He pointed out that since fluoride comes as a waste product from smokestack scrubbers, it is contaminated with "lead, arsenic and radium, all of them carcinogenic." He added that fluoridated cities have twice the hip fractures than elsewhere and fluoride is "altering the basic architecture of human bones."

Fluorosis

Fluoride affects the teeth by changing the structure of the calcium crystals, the building blocks of the teeth. If fluoride is present when the teeth are formed (ages 0 - 15), it will be found throughout the enamel. That is why the fluoride proponents want kids exposed to fluoride from birth until all the teeth are formed.

If too much fluoride is present during the formation of a tooth, it will show fluorosis, which appears as a "mottling" of the color of the tooth, a non-uniform white haze over the tooth that makes it look chalky. Fluoride can also cause splotchy areas of intense white. If you live in an area that has fluoridated water, look at the teeth of a couple of teenagers; most will show signs of

387

fluorosis because it is common in areas where the water is fluoridated. As the amount of fluoride exposure increases, the white areas become larger and more unattractive. With enough fluoride, the enamel changes and the teeth become dark and brittle. Dark, unattractive teeth is not a look most people want.

Fluoride Drops For Children

Hopefully, the use of fluoride drops and tablets for children may soon be a thing of the past. Even though these prescription drugs have been in use for years, it seems that no one ever did the required studies to show them to be safe and effective. The FDA let them be sold without any positive studies, which is a violation of the FDA's own rules. This is an example of how the FDA can be selective in applying its rules. Parents should avoid using these products.

Fluoridated Toothpaste

Most people are currently using toothpaste that contains fluoride, because all commercial toothpaste has gotten on the fluoride bandwagon so they can get the ADA "Seal of Acceptance." That relationship leaves no other commercial choices. (However, using baking soda is a natural way to avoid fluoridated toothpaste.) The danger for children using fluoridated toothpaste is similar to that of fluoride treatments. Since babies are born with a sucking reflex, they suck in food and will do the same with toothpaste. Children can swallow too much fluoride in toothpaste, (There may not be such a thing as sucking in too little fluoride.) Another reason why so many people have fluorosed teeth.

The easiest way to avoid this swallowing problem is not to let children three and under use toothpaste. If you do allow your child to use toothpaste, use the smallest amount that you, not the child, can put on the toothbrush. Of course, if the child does not eat and drink sugar, you have little need to worry about plaque and decay.

Fluoride Treatments

It is an accepted practice in the United States to give fluoride treatments to children under the age of 18 years.

These treatments were originally given only to children who were at risk for decay, but gradually, dentists began to give the treatments to almost every child, figuring it could do no harm and might do some good. Of course, the fact that it was a good way to add thousands of dollars in profits to their practice every year had nothing to do with it.

The sweet-tasting, flavored fluoride gel is placed in a disposable tray and put in the child's mouth, who is then told to chew with the tray in place to force the gel between the teeth. But this treatment has been fatal at least once because small children still have the sucking reflex. One very young child who was given a fluoride treatment swallowed most of it. Later that day he was taken to a hospital but, not soon enough to get the fatal dose of fluoride out of his system.

Is that a risk that should stop you from having fluoride treatments done to your children? It should be if they are under age six. Other children should only have these treatments if they are getting decay, which they only get if they are not eating right. One of the last fluoride treatments in my practice was done about 20 years ago on one of my own children. Although he was around 12 years old, he still swallowed so much fluoride that he threw up. Maybe he was lucky he reacted by ejecting the poison, although at the time that was not my first thought!

Fluoride Treatment For Dogs

Veterinarians have jumped on the profit-making fluoride treatments by giving them to our pets, a terrible disservice which you should never allow. To begin with, animals would never get any cavities unless they are fed the same junk food we feed ourselves. So even if fluoride was a good idea for humans, it would not be a good idea for pets. Any vet who uses such questionable treatment as fluoride treatment for dogs should be watched closely for other worthless recommendations whose principle purpose is to separate us from our money.

Fluoride Rinses

If fluoride rinses are effective, and new studies cast doubt on that claim, they are only needed by people who are abusing their teeth with lousy diets. Is the answer to tooth decay a mouth rinse with a toxic chemical or a modification of the diet which is the real cause of the damage? Of course, it is the latter, but most people are more willing to risk the toxic chemical if they can continue their poor eating habits. If a person chooses to continue the habits that cause the problem, all the fluoride rinse in the world will not stop the inevitable. If the behavior is corrected so damage is not being done, then the rinses will not be needed, even if they did work.

In many areas the public health nurses or dental hygienists give fluoride rinses to schoolchildren. However, this practice is illegal because they are dispensing a prescription drug without a license. Prescription drugs can only be ordered by a doctor for a specific person; therefore, they cannot legally be given to large groups, even if parents sign a permission slip. Still, fluoride rinses are given to millions of children every year because the local public health departments, under the influence of the ADA, think it is a good idea.

Fluoride And Cancer

The incidence of decay is higher in many adults than it is in children. Tooth decay, still the most common disease in America, has begun to have a delayed onset. Up to 50 percent of the senior population has root decay, for example: the dental profession's predictable response is to recommend that adults get more fluoride. Now many dentists recommend fluoride treatments for adults, as well as for children. It is a new "profit center" for dental practices.

But do we not get enough exposure to fluorides as it is? It is in our water, our food, our drinks, and our toothpaste. It was once proposed to add it to our milk. How much additional exposure could we possibly need when the amount we are currently receiving does not appear effective? Twice as much? Four times as much? A HUNDRED TIMES?

Congressional Fluoride Study

A continuing controversy has been taking place over the use of fluoride in the drinking water since it was first proposed after World War II. To end the controversy, Congress, in the early 1980's, authorized a study to find out once and for all whether fluoride causes cancer. No one seemed to work quickly on the project, as it took several years to set up the study and another 10 years to get the data. Finally, the results were published: they showed that fluoride does cause cancer. Did the FDA order an end to water fluoridation? No, instead it recommended that the safety limit of fluoride in water be doubled!

The study was attacked, not scientifically, but politically. The media were used by the pro-fluoridationists when they issued a report saying that the study was wrong and that fluoride is safe, after all. As a result, the public became more confused. Then, to further quell the critics and reassure the public, came the inevitable call for more studies. Nothing has changed including the increased death rate.

In one case a healthy 28-year-old construction worker hit his leg. At first it seemed only to be bruised, but it did not heal. He then went to see his doctor who found an osteosarcoma, a rare bone cancer, the type of cancer found in the Congressional fluoride study. Within six weeks the patient was dead! It was sad to see a healthy young man succumb to cancer so quickly.

Was this man's cancer caused by fluoride? No one can say, but osteosarcomas are virtually nonexistent in non-fluoridated areas. Can we tell his loved ones that we are doing "another study?" Would they be comforted if they knew that fluoride may save a few teeth from getting cavities that are entirely preventable if people ate a more nutritious diet? How many more senseless deaths are we willing to tolerate to eat and drink sugar? The time for studies is before we use the public as guinea pigs, not after!

International Use of Fluoride

Following is a list of the countries that currently approve the use of fluoride in the public water supply and the percentage of the population who get fluoridated water:

Country	% of population (in millions)	Actual number of people
Australia	66	10.5
Canada	50	13.0
(Former)Czechoslovakia	20	3.0
(Former) East Germany	9	1.5
Finland	1.5	0.07
Ireland	50	1.75
New Zealand	66	2.2
Spain	1	3.0
Switzerland	4	0.26
United Kingdom	9	5.1
United States	50	122.0
(Former) USSR	15	42.6

The total number of people in the world with fluoride in their drinking water is approximately 205 million, only four percent of the world population. In addition, the numbers from the former communist countries may be questionable, even if accurate, but show that 60 percent of all people drinking fluoridated water are Americans.

The list of countries without fluoridation is long. To the people in these countries we must add the people spared from fluoridation in countries that use it. Many of these non-fluoridated countries have a history of socialized medicine; countries you expect would be most likely to use a program to save them money. Countries such as Sweden, Norway, and Denmark do not offer any fluoridation to their people. Other major industrialized countries which do not promote fluoridation are Austria, Bulgaria, France Greece, Hungary, Italy, Japan, Portugal, and Romania. Third world countries with huge populations, such as China, Egypt, India, Indonesia, and Turkey are also spared fluoridation. Can you believe that a country like Japan would not introduce fluoridation if they had any knowledge that it would be in the public good?

Protecting Reputations, Not The Public

Many American public health officials, including the ADA, have staked their reputations on the value and safety of fluoride. Nothing is more tenacious than bureaucrats trying to protect their reputation. Smaller countries seem more willing to stop dangerous public health programs. Both the former West Germany and the Netherlands abandoned fluoridation after decades of experimentation.

This overwhelming avoidance of fluoridation should make us wonder what they know that our public health officials are keeping from us. The concept of fluoridation has been actively promoted by American public health officials for over 50 years, yet most every other country has declined to subject their people to this unquestionably dangerous practice. America has a history of denying publication of any anti-fluoride papers. Scientists who have tried to oppose fluoridation do so at the risk of loss of position and funding. Squelching dissent is a tool of the powerful to maintain their questionable practices from the light of truth and open debate. In this manner they believe they can keep the public ignorant. Fortunately, the light of truth is impossible to deny and will eventually come out. It is sad that so many will suffer because of the delay.

Conclusion

How do people's teeth in other countries survive when they do not have the "advantage" of being drenched in fluorides? How do the billions of other mammals on earth survive without decay when they do not drink fluoridated water? Why has decay remained a problem in America and other Western countries if fluorides truly prevented decay? Will there ever come a time when humans eat the foods to nourish them instead of those that hurt them?

Our diet is so bad that it actually causes our living body to decay while we are alive. It should shock you to know what we are doing to ourselves. The new food labels help show us what is in our processed foods so the sugars are not as hidden as they once were. But knowing is different than acting on that knowledge. When the average American eats two and a half pounds of sugar per week, we are consuming 10 to 15 times the sugar our ancestors did a hundred years ago. Unfortunately, the high sugar consumption seems to be getting worse.

We need to quit thinking in terms of symptoms, such as decay, and begin to think about causes, such as consuming too much sugar. We value our health so little that we sacrifice it for a "taste of honey." We become so oriented toward momentary pleasures that we are willing to give up our teeth for a bottle of carbonated sugar water. If we continue in this direction, all the dentists in the world cannot save us from ourselves!

17

OTHER DANGERS

Avoiding Exposure To Metals

The mouth is not the only way toxic metals can enter the body. We get many metals in our food and drinks; others we absorb through our skin or by smoking. Every inorganic, metal-containing molecule we absorb, no matter what the source, is either eliminated by the body or stored for future elimination. Toxic metals are all poisonous to us to one degree or another, so it is best that we reduce our exposure to pure metals as much as possible.

For instance, to reduce aluminum exposure, we should avoid aluminum cookware, aluminum cans and anti-perspirants (not deodorants). To reduce exposure to chromium and nickel, we must avoid stainless steel, such as cookware and watch bands (use leather instead) and watch backs (cover with tape). Other options can help us avoid these and other exposures to toxic metals.

It is up to each of us to be aware that our bodies are from the "Stone Age" and were not designed to handle the toxins which inundate us in our modern society. Even when we are diligent, we face much exposure, so any exposure that we can avoid, we must. It was not that long ago that our meals were cooked in safe iron pots and pans, that men wore pocket watches they wound daily, or our noses were not so quickly offended if someone smelled less than freshly scrubbed. We need to be ever diligent in our efforts to avoid needless metal contamination.

Damage Is Related

People tend to live day to day without considering the accumulating damage done to their bodies from bad habits, damage which they must live with when older, if they survive. It is easy to rationalize bad habits when we are young because young, people think of themselves as immortal. When we are young, it is hard to relate to the person we will become in our forties and beyond. But it is that person who must live or die by those health habits we choose now. It is too late to quit smoking on the way to have lung surgery or to give up carbonated beverages when you are scheduled for surgery to have your teeth removed. We must take responsibility for our long-term health starting today.

Young people tend to discount advice from people their parents' age because "they can't possibly understand what we're going through." For example, ex-smokers, emphysema sufferers, and terminal lung cancer patients seemingly have little influence in preventing teens from beginning the smoking habit. The message kids seem to get from their cultural heroes who have overcome addictions is not that they should keep from starting a bad habit, rather that they can follow the same behavior and quit when they get in trouble.

Early Damage

A truth young people are not told or do not understand is that any drug habit, legal or illegal, which they begin before their bodies are mature, will cause damage quicker and with longer-lasting effects than one started later in life. A person who begins drinking at age 16 may become an alcoholic at age 21, even if he does not drink a lot. The same person, if he began drinking at 21, may never become an alcoholic, even though he consumes similar or even greater quantities over longer periods of time. Young women seem to be even more susceptible to early damage than young men. Teens believe adults are trying to keep them from enjoying the "good stuff." Yet it really is true that their bodies are not ready to be "abused."

This concept applies to sugar. The longer children can be kept from eating candy and soft drinks, the healthier they will be and the less likely they will be to crave non-nutritious foods that will hurt them. It is much better to show love with a kind word or a hug than to give a sugar treat. Sugar can quickly turn from a "fun food" to a metabolic poison. Every cavity a child has is a direct result of the poor food choices of their parents.

Alcohol

The use of alcohol has both direct and indirect effects on oral health. Alcohol use is directly associated with an increase in oral cancers. One of the effects of alcohol is to dry living tissue by driving out water, which is how tissue specimens are preserved in a laboratory. This chronic irritation of the oral tissues may lead to tissue damage, which may allow the cancers to form.

The secondary effect of heavy alcohol use is to upset the natural functions of vitamins and minerals. Alcohol depletes the body of the B vitamins needed for nerve function. Alcohol also depresses the appetite, discouraging alcoholics from eating well, which further reduces nutrition and therefore, limits the body's ability to heal itself. Their mouth, as well as their whole body, shows the effects of this induced malnutrition, because routine damage cannot be repaired without the proper nutrients. Alcohol is really a supercharged form of sugar, and its effects on the body are the same as sugar except greatly exaggerated.

A dentist can tell a heavy drinker by his dehydrated look. When he is both a drinker and a smoker, chances that his teeth will last his whole life are less than for most other groups. An alcoholic however, is not concerned. Why would someone worry about his teeth lasting another 10 years when all he really cares about is when he will get his next drink? Until heavy drinkers (and smokers) change their personal priorities, a dentist's concern for their oral health is wasted.

Tobacco

If you stopped smoking, and cigarettes were banned, ninety-five percent of lung cancer would go away.

Homer Twigg,
Assistant Professor
Indiana University School of Medicine

It seems that the human race cannot be content without vices, and tobacco is one of its favorites. Currently, tobacco is under siege because of the serious health problems it causes. The tide against tobacco use is rising. At this writing, the truth about how tobacco companies have been using additives in their tobaccos, possibly even adding or "adjusting" the nicotine levels to increase addiction, is being revealed.

Tobacco has always had critics, just as mercury in fillings has always been opposed by some dentists, but smoking never became so abused until American ingenuity was applied. Smoking a pipe at the village pub while discussing the weather is far different than smoking a pack of the manufactured tubes of tobacco called cigarettes used today.

The cancer connection was first mentioned in the popular press in the *Reader's Digest* in the 1920's. Seventy-five years later, 25 percent of adults are still smoking (that's FIFTY MILLION people!), and smoking is increasing among teens. It would seem that having tens of thousands premature deaths annually from smoking would be an incentive for every smoker to quit. After all, that is many times more deaths than the number of people killed by guns.

Until the turn of the century chewing tobacco was the most popular form of tobacco. Spittoons were everywhere. There was so much spitting on the sidewalks that ordinances prohibiting it were passed. While normal hygiene was a factor, the real reason was the discovery that tuberculosis was found to be carried in the saliva, and this was an attempt to help stop the spread of the disease. Today, if you watch a professional baseball game, you will see enough spitting around home plate to kill all the grass! These players serve as bad examples for our youth to glamorize and may account for the increase use of both chewing tobacco and snuff. Round tins in the hip pocket of our teen boys tell everyone how "cool" it is to use snuff.

The truth is that all three tobacco habits—smoking, chewing, and using snuff—are terrible from every aspect. From the dental point of view these habits are not only damaging, but can sometimes be disfiguring and even fatal. Snuff, for example, damages the gums and bone because it causes a chemical bump on the cheek and gums as the sensitive tissue tries to protect itself from the toxins. The increase in oral cancers correlates with the increase in the use of these "smokeless" tobaccos.

Since alcohol also contributes to oral cancer, and tobacco and alcohol are frequently used together, many users are getting a double whammy. The total incidence of oral cancers is about 50,000 cases per year with 8,000 deaths. Surgeries to remove some of these cancers are traumatic and destroy the victim's quality of life.

Gum Damage

Smoking is also a major cause of gum problems. The media emphasizes cancer and emphysema, but these problems do not affect every smoker. The resulting gum problems, however do affect anyone who smokes. More teeth are lost due to gum problems than any other single problem, and smoking is a main culprit. The damage may be due to an induced scurvy (lack of vitamin C) caused by the toxic products in the smoke. Smoke contains many free radicals (chemically active substances which can damage normal molecules when they combine with them), which the body tries to neutralize with vitamin C. But a pack of cigarettes quickly uses up the vitamin C in the average person. Most smokers are, therefore, in a chronic state of vitamin C deficiency, which happens to be the definition of scurvy. A deficiency of vitamin C also means that the other normal functions of this vitamin cannot be performed.

Taking extra vitamin C, at least a 1000 mg a day, is helpful, but not as much as quitting smoking. Smokers' gums tend to be soft and spongy. Bleeding and swelling are common. A dentist can tell a smoker by a glance at his gums. When a person quits, these symptoms reverse and the gums can return to a more healthy condition without the person changing lifestyle.

The chances for serious gum problems are much higher for smokers than for non-smokers. Since gum problems are common, even among non-smokers, smokers can expect a 100 percent incidence of gum disease. The only escape is quitting. It is sad to tell smokers that they are likely to lose all their teeth as a result of the damage done by smoking. It is sadder still to see that knowing this, does not seem to stop any of them from smoking. If the chance of dying from lung cancer or emphysema does not stop them, losing their teeth certainly will not!

Chewing Tobacco

Chewing tobacco is gross to everyone, even the chewer, so gross that it should be grounds for divorce. If non-chewing men had to kiss women who chewed tobacco, it would be! Even though this form of tobacco does not seem to be as damaging as smoking and snuff, it does present its own problems. Tobacco leaves contain fine particles of silica picked up from the soil. Most of us call silica "sand." Now what do you think would happen if you chewed sand—maybe wear the enamel on the top of the teeth? That is exactly what happens to tobacco chewers. Chewing tobacco wears the teeth flat like millstones. A certain amount of wearing is good for teeth, as is seen in the non-decayed teeth of primitive tribes and skulls that predate the modem era. The wearing of the molars is even common today in most countries, where the food is not as soft as ours, and helps keep the tops of the teeth polished so smooth that decay is rare.

However, this wear often becomes excessive with tobacco chewers. Also, if mercury fillings are present on the chewing surfaces, chewing tobacco wears the fillings even more than it wears the enamel, thus exposing chewers to more mercury entering their bodies.

Tobacco chewers' gum problems are usually less severe than with the users of other types of tobacco. An additional concern is that chewers tend to be in the group that visits dentists the least, as they seem to be more independent, self-sufficient types of men, such as farmers. Maybe farmers have more places to spit than bankers!

Remember, one or more of the health problems caused by smoking will affect every smoker. If you smoke, can you climb a flight of stairs without getting out of breath? Do you wheeze when you breathe even without exertion? If so, you will some day have to pull a bottle of oxygen around with you, so you can go to the store. Loss of teeth and premature death should be enough of an incentive to convince anyone to quit smoking. If you use tobacco, please do everyone, particularly yourself, a favor and quit. Millions of others have already quit, and they were not as smart or as strong-willed as you. If they could quit, so can you. If you will not do it for yourself, then do it to aggravate the tobacco companies, which loves the profits, and the government, which loves tobacco taxes.

18

WHAT YOU CAN DO

How To Avoid Dental Problems And Keep Your Teeth For A Lifetime

Many simple methods can be used to avoid dental problems that each of us can use and teach our children and grandchildren. The conventional wisdom is to brush and floss twice a day, see your dentist twice a year, and drink fluoridated water. Occasionally, you may also hear advice about cutting down on the sugar. It would be nice if avoiding dental problems were that simple, so that most Americans would have complete sets of undamaged teeth.

Unfortunately, most Americans have many dental problems, including mouths full of dental work, crowded and crooked teeth, gum problems, routinely missing teeth, and even no teeth at all. Since these problems affect the vast majority of Americans from children on up, the "conventional wisdom" must be wrong. Fortunately, has the ability every person to control or eliminate those factors that are damaging to oral health and to take action to improve it. It is much less costly to prevent the problems than to fix them after they occur. As an added plus, it is more comfortable not to have to endure dental work.

A Typical Example

A typical example of how careless people can be about taking care of their teeth is the case of a 46-year-old man who went to the dentist because he had a tooth that hurt. His complaint was that his "filling fell out." As is routinely true, the filling did not fall out, but a piece of tooth had broken off after it was undermined by decay. The patient had 22 teeth (the best mouths usually have only 28 after the wisdom teeth have been removed, so 22 teeth is not unusual). He only had two with fillings and no other cavities in the remaining teeth, which is far above average.

Part of this patient's problem was that he had not been to a dentist in years and could not remember the last time he had had his teeth cleaned, a clear indication of how little he valued his teeth or professional care. A large percentage of Americans go to the dentist only when they have a "problem," which means they go when the problem becomes so bad they can no longer ignore it.

That was the case with this patient. His X-ray showed a large cavity and in addition, a lot of damage to the bone supporting the decayed tooth, which meant that the tooth had to be extracted. However, the patient was not surprised or worried. He said, "They won't last much longer anyway," because his mindset was that people lose their teeth when they get older. In his case it was a self-fulfilling prophecy because there was such widespread damage to the bone supporting his remaining teeth that no amount of good intentions, changed habits, or heroic dental work could stop the eventual loss of his teeth. So much deterioration at such a young age is not uncommon, particularly among blue-collar men who smoke.

Key Factors

The key factors that destroyed the bone in this patient's mouth and caused his teeth to drift apart were entirely within his control. Smoking, poor nutrition (scurvy), lack of seeking even minimal professional care, and his mindset that any preventative care is a waste of time and money because he will loose his teeth anyway, all added up to a certain loss of his teeth. Unfortunately, he is not alone in either his choice of self-destructive habits or his self-defeating mindset. We all know people who would greatly benefit from a change in certain habits, even ourselves.

Health is produced only by healthful living.
Unknown

Keys To Maintaining A Healthy Mouth

What can you do to maintain a healthier mouth? Read through the following suggestions and rate yourself on a scale of one to ten, with one being "very poor" and ten being "very good". This is a secret test; no one else has to know the results. Sometimes, we are afraid of actually checking to see how far we are from where we should be, but you need to know where you are before you can begin to improve.

1) GET NECESSARY NUTRIENTS

"Boring, boring, boring. Don't lecture me on what to eat. I eat what I like!" is a typical response to anyone discussing nutrition. Could it be that getting nutritional advice makes us feel like children again? "Eat your brussel sprouts; they're good for you!" Our mothers told us. We all have childhood memories of being forced to eat something that to this day we refuse to eat.

407

And even though we are adults now and should know how to eat right, we act as if we neither know nor care even though nutrition underlies our health and longevity. We all could dramatically improve the quality of our diet beginning today. Continual exposure to good information on what will nourish our bodies helps remind us that we control our choices and can chose to do better today than yesterday.

The best place to begin is before the beginning. A healthy girl who matures into a healthy woman has a good chance to having healthy eggs, which after fertilization by sperm from an equally healthy man, will have the best chance to develop into a healthy baby. This newborn baby should have its mother's milk, as nature intended, for as long as possible to give the growing child the best possible start. As the child gets older, he needs to get as many fresh vegetables and fruits as possible. These foods, which can be eaten raw or only lightly cooked, will greatly help in the building of the growing body, which, in turn will strongly influence the health of the adult. Proper eating habits learned in childhood will continue into adulthood, AS WILL POOR EATING HABITS. Avoid giving children high-fat snacks, sugary candy and soft drinks. If a child grows up without drinking soft drinks, he will not use them much as an adult. On the other hand, a child raised on potato chips, candy bars, and soft drinks will not become a healthy eater as an adult without extraordinary effort.

It is the parents' and grandparents' responsibility to help children grow as healthy as possible by guiding them to eat the better foods. Expect them to eat better food; demand that they eat better food. Do not let the children choose poor foods just because they come with a toy! Remember, healthy children have healthy teeth.

As an adult, you need to continue eating as much fresh, whole food as possible. Remember, a whole food is an apple, not an apple pie. A good rule to follow is to eat a minimum of five to seven servings of fruits and vegetables each day. How many did you have yesterday? Consuming this many servings a day may seem impossible for many "meat and potato" eaters, but it can be done. Instead of that second doughnut, eat an orange with your breakfast. (Orange juice doesn't count!) For a mid-morning snack, have a banana. At night, cut a wedge of cabbage and eat it raw. Have bags of celery, carrots, broccoli, and cauliflower cut into relish tray sizes for snacks during TV viewing. Eating these five servings a day would vastly improve the health of tens of millions of people.

ADDITIONAL VITAMINS AND MINERALS

As an adjunct most people would benefit from taking some additional nutritional support in the form of vitamin and mineral tablets. Overwhelming evidence proves that most of us are overfed and undernourished, meaning we get plenty of sugar, fat and protein but too little of the essential nutrients, such as certain vitamins and minerals. While individual requirements vary, certain minimums are needed, and they exceed the government's minimum daily requirements. By the name alone, these are only minimum requirements, meant to keep a person from a deficiency, such as having scurvy from getting too little vitamin C. Sick people need five to seven times as much of these nutrients, as do pregnant women and older people who have more problems with digestion. Actually, we have very few really well nourished people in our country.

No one can go wrong taking daily the following supplements: Vitamin C 1000-3000mg, magnesium 300mg, beta carotene 15mg, a B-50 complex, co-enzyme Q-10 100mg, and calcium 1000mg, along with a trace mineral supplement that supplies manganese, chromium, selenium, and zinc. A reasonable amount of added fiber will help replace the natural fiber lacking in our diet. Even with seven servings of fruits and vegetables, most of us will be below the recommended 30 grams of fiber per day. Fiber is important because it helps move waste products out of the body, including mercury.

2) DO THOROUGH DAILY DENTAL CARE:

It is important to spend a reasonable amount of time cleaning your teeth, including flossing. Brushing and flossing after meals are still recommended, but many patients tell their dentists that they have just brushed, while plaque is thick on their front teeth. Although brushing after meals is a good guideline for all to follow, the amount of time needed for proper cleaning depends on the diet. People who only eat fruits and vegetables will not have much plaque growth because natural, whole foods do not feed plaque, and in addition, these type foods clean our teeth while we chew.

Use your gums as an indicator of whether you are doing a good job cleaning your mouth. If your gums bleed when you thoroughly clean your teeth and gums, then you need to work harder on your daily cleaning regimen and your diet. Using baking soda right out of the box as a dentifrice, instead of toothpaste, is a good place to start. Once you are used to its salty taste rather than the sugary toothpaste taste, it will become a pleasant habit. Baking soda also neutralizes acids produced by plaque, helping keep the mouth near a neutral pH. Using hydrogen peroxide may also help to combat gum infection. (Avoid peroxide if you have metals in your mouth.)

3) AVOID BAD HABIT:

Habits damaging to your body also damage you mouth. The most damaging habit is smoking. Much of smoking's bad effects are due to our bodies needing more vitamins, particularly vitamin C, to protect us from its toxins. Another bad habit, excessive drinking (more than two drinks per day), has a similar effect of "using up" vitamins, particularly vitamin B-complex. Alcohol also dehydrates (takes water out of) the tissues. Both of these habits are strongly associated with oral cancers, as is the use of "smokeless" tobacco, which has a high association with oral cancers because of the chronic irritation it causes.

4) AVOID ACCIDENTS:

It is common to see a young person with a front tooth chipped from an accident that occurred while playing sports, but many are from when someone else was "playing around." For instance, when patients are asked how their front tooth got chipped they say, "My brother hit me with a rock," or "Someone pushed me while I was drinking from a fountain." These chips can lead to fillings, crowns, root-canals, tooth loss, and various replacements. All these dental problems could be avoided if the accident is avoided.

Chipped front teeth are most common in children who have overbites because their teeth are in a more vulnerable position. Some of these overbites are caused by food allergies that begin in infancy (commonly cow's milk) that result in breathing problems, which in turn distort the shape of the mouth. Parents and pediatricians need to be aware of these symptoms to help the children avoid problems by catching them early. If an overbite develops, have it corrected at the earliest age possible to reduce the threat of accidents to the front teeth. Many children chip their front teeth falling off their bikes, which may be reduced with the increase in the use of bike helmets.

A common cause of dental damage in adults is car accidents. In addition, many men damage their front teeth in accidents that occur while handling tools or playing sports. The toothless smile of a hockey team is a running joke. Since most organized sports require a mouth protector to be used injuries often happen during "pickup" games.

5) *EXERCISE:* EXERCISE?

How do you exercise the mouth? You do it by chewing. It is important that we chew to stimulate bone density around the teeth, promote salivary flow which contains digestive enzymes, and improve the food's digestibility by breaking it into tiny pieces. Chewing is a good habit to teach children, who prefer soft foods that are easily swallowed, particularly if they have a soft drink to wash them down. Remember, it is not our job to make it easy for children to eat, only to provide nourishing, health-promoting foods.

Exercising the whole body is also good for the teeth. Bone stressed by exercise becomes harder and stronger, including the bone around your teeth. If the calcium mechanisms work as they should, our bodies conserve our calcium supply. Without exercise, we lose calcium, some through the saliva, which can end up on our teeth as tartar deposits. So exercise can really help keep your teeth clean.

6) *GET GOOD DENTAL CARE*

In the absence of decay, caused by a poor diet, little professional care is really necessary. An occasional cleaning may be a good idea, but such treatment is usually needed less often than every six months. With good habits, you might only need one cleaning every several years or maybe never. Many dentists find that with proper care they do not need to get their own teeth cleaned. Every dentist knows of patients they see who could go years without needing a professional cleaning (but they get one anyway!).

Although you may not require a professional cleaning, you still need to visit a dentist because even highly motivated people can develop unseen problems. It is important to have a set of bitewing X-rays taken to check for hidden decay and to monitor the health of the bone around the teeth. While bitewing X-rays are routinely done every year, in a healthy person with a clean mouth, every two years would be adequate. To look for other hidden problems in the whole mouth area, a panoramic X-ray should be taken every five years. A full-mouth series of X-rays is not recommended because it requires approximately 16 X-rays and still does not reach all the areas a panoramic X-ray reaches. New imaging techniques are becoming available coupling computers and X-ray machines that hold the promise of improved images while reducing the total amount of radiation necessary.

Replacement of failing dental work and proper placing of new dental work, following the guidelines found in this book, are important. The replacement of poorly done dental work and the removal of toxic dental materials should be done before they cause major immune problems. If no decay occurs, a tooth will not need dental work, and avoiding the need for dental work is the safest path.

7) HAVE THE PROPER MIND SET:

It is important to have a realistic view of what oral health is and how it can be achieved. The fact that our parents have lost their teeth does not mean we must to lose ours. It is more likely that we can identify specific eating and other health habits that caused our parents to lose their teeth. Poor teeth are not usually a genetic problem but rather the result of our following our parents' poor example in all the above categories. We do not need to condemn our parents for what they did; we must assume they did the best they knew how at the time. We can build on the good things they did and add things that we have learned.

This view also works the other way, in that many good things parents do are rejected by their children as "old-fashioned." In many instances the "old ways" are closer to nature and healthier. Except for infectious diseases, our forefathers were very healthy. The average modern man would be hard-pressed to match our "caveman" ancestors in strength and stamina. Dentally, they did not have any decay even without the availability of fluoridated toothpaste and electric toothbrushes.

Many people believe they will repeat their parents' experience of losing all their teeth. Unfortunately, if they think they are doomed, then they may well be. Our thinking tends to lead us to fulfill our thoughts. In this case the notion,"I think, therefore I am," becomes, "I think I will lose my teeth, therefore I will!" But we have the power to change our future by thinking, "I won't repeat the bad habits that caused my parents to lose their teeth; therefore I'll keep my teeth for my whole life."

It is a matter of self-discipline to do the things we know are good for us in spite of all the time and advertising pressures we face. We do not have to yield the control of our minds to TV commercials that want us to behave in ways that will profit them and hurt us. We can take control of our future any time we want, for instance, RIGHT NOW!

19

THE SPECTRE OF HIV/AIDS

The Impact of HIV/Aids on Dentistry

The fear of AIDS is growing; no one knows how far the disease will go before it reaches its limit of destruction. There is no acknowledged way to stop the spread of the disease, except celibacy or an HIV-free monogamous relationship. Even these ways may not be enough protection, because the blood supply is not 100 percent safe and nonsexual means of transmission also exist. Even though HIV is the most studied virus ever, no headway is being made by traditional medicine toward a vaccination or cure.

Some people may have stopped going to the dentist because of the fear of catching the virus. The highly publicized AIDS cases linked to the Florida dentist, Dr. Acer, have made people hesitate to get treatment. No one blames people for being cautious. However, the fact is, the risk of being infected with HIV in a dental office is extremely remote to the point of not being a risk at all. The real risk is that the dentist will catch something from a patient, be it HIV, hepatitis, or even a common cold.

The scientific community has suspected that dentists might be at risk of contracting HIV from their patients, ever since the virus was identified. The first group at risk were dentists in the San Francisco area, because they were being exposed before anyone knew of the disease and could take precautions; so far this has not been reported to have happened. Nevertheless, the precautions dentists now take to protect themselves have increased dramatically because of their vulnerability. These precautions also protect you, the patient.

Dr. Acer

What of Dr. Acer's patients in Florida? As of now, no one has identified any clinical way they could have been accidentally infected by him. Although Dr. Acer had been accused of deliberately infecting them, it is more likely that they got infected from other sources. It is difficult to imagine anyone in his right mind, particularly a healthcare professional, doing something so evil as deliberately infecting innocent people. It has also been shown that in spite of their denials, each of his patients that had HIV could have gotten infected in more "normal" ways.

Other Considerations

First of all, considering the current levels of HIV in our population, the percentage of Dr. Acer's HIV-positive patients corresponds to the expected levels. In other words, a small proportion of any dentist's patients may be HIV-positive, more so in urban areas. Additionally, the strain of the HIV with which Dr. Acer's patients were infected did not exactly match his virus, but did match other strains in that area. During investigations each person who claimed to have been infected by Dr. Acer was shown to have had other possible exposures. It is quite possible that he did not cause a single one of these patients to contract HIV; if that is true, he has been slandered, and the dental profession has been unduly attacked. The more reasonable facts about HIV and dentistry have not received much attention because it is much more sensational and convenient to blame Dr. Acer. But finally, in June 1994, these other possibilities were discussed on a "*60 Minutes*" TV segment. Why would the ADA and The Centers for Disease Control (CDC) be so quick to blame Dr. Acer, if he may not have been at fault? It is possible that these entities have let the idea that he deliberately infected his patients go unchallenged because it is in their best interest to do so. If people think Dr. Acer infected his patients, deliberately then the sterilizing standards of "Universal Precautions" will not be questioned (see "Universal Precautions"). While the current sterilizing standards are good if correctly followed, they were not commonly used when these patients contracted HIV.

Several of Dr. Acer's patients have been paid "out of court" to settle lawsuits. It was the insurance companies' decision that it would cost less to pay off the claims than to fight. Several of Dr. Acer's other patients may not get anything because all the money available was taken by the first people to file suit. The whole situation was a matter of solving a publicity nightmare as quickly as possible with the least cost and the fewest questions raised by the media and the public. Better to settle than to fight to protect the dentist's reputation. Anyway, he was already dead and had become a convenient scapegoat. Unfortunately, all of Dr. Acer's HIV-positive patients will ultimately die, and the attention these cases received has only raised that much more fear among the public.

While it is possible that Dr. Acer did deliberately infect his patients, it is more likely that he was innocent of any wrongdoing. If his sterilization techniques were not perfect, they were still better than those many other dentists were using at the time. If the spread of HIV were easily possible in a dental office, many other cases would have surfaced by now. Until there is definite proof that Dr. Acer acted improperly, he has the right, even in death, to be judged "innocent until proven guilty."

Purposes of Sterilization

The purpose of sterilization is to stop the transmission of germs from the last patient to the healthcare team and the next patient, but not to protect the patient from the dentist. For the dentist to be a threat to the patient, he would first have to be infected and have an open, uncovered, bleeding wound of some type. Then, the patient would also have to have an open wound. Finally, the blood from the dentist would have to get in the patient's wound. While that sequence could happen, it is highly unlikely to improbable. Imagine how that sequence could take place: During an extraction the dentist slips and a scalpel cuts a finger. Some blood leaks through the glove and gets into an open wound in the patient's mouth. This accident could happen, but only rarely. Ask your dentist if he has ever been cut with a scalpel or other instrument. He will probably say he has never been cut and does not know of any dentist who has. If the Florida dentist managed to cut himself six or more times in a year or two, he would have to be the clumsiest dentist that ever lived!

Contaminated Needles

The only common source of possible contamination is with a needle stick when a used needle accidentally penetrates another person's skin. If a dentist happens to stick himself before injecting a patient, he knows enough to stop; first, to treat himself and

418

second, to get rid of the contaminated needle. No dentist would continue to use the same needle! Dentists do not have needle stick accidents that often, particularly today, when strict precautions are used.

If Dr. Acer was clumsy and did stick himself with a needle and then used it on patients, he would have violated many standard procedures. It is more likely that the dentist would get a needle stick after injecting the patient, not before. If a needle stick accident did happen, still no infection may result because this is not an effective way to transmit HIV. It is estimated that the odds are 300 to 1 that a needle stick will transmit HIV from one person to another. If this is true, that would mean that Dr. Acer would have had to have accidentally stick himself first, then a patient, hundreds and hundreds of times to contaminate six patients. No one is that clumsy!

Should you be afraid of getting any infection in a dental office? No! Should you be cautious? Yes! Make sure your dentist practices universal precautions, so your risk is virtually zero. Even if the dentist has HIV (knowingly or unknowingly), your risk is still virtually zero. That stated position of the CDC is probably correct, since if HIV contraction were a risk in a dental office, many more such clusters of HIV-infected patients would have appeared by now.

HIV-Infected Doctors

If the public so desired and lobbied hard to enact new laws, a dentist or physician with HIV could be removed from active practice. An HIV screening of all health professionals could be done every three or six months to detect the virus. If a dentist or any other type of doctor were found to be positive, then a previously established disability insurance program would allow him to retire and draw disability income.

Now, most dentists who have HIV must continue work or go bankrupt. Occasionally, when a professional can no longer work due to HIV/AIDS, his disability insurance may pay him but no promises are made by the insurance companies, thus forcing dentists to keep working as long as they can or face financial ruin. Thus, doctors are afraid to be tested because the public would force them from practice.

Most dentists carry disability insurance to protect them from loss of income due to a disabling injury or illness, including mental illness. However, the insurance companies are reluctant to pay disability for HIV unless it can be proven it was contracted at work that the dentist may have caught HIV from sources other than through a patient, a false worry because other types of disability do not have to be work-related. For example, if a dentist is disabled in a car accident, his insurance is valid.

If the government's position were that HIV infection were a disability for doctors, then they could collect under their policies. Unfortunately, the government says that it is okay for an HIV-carrying professional to work on patients because the odds are that he will not transmit the virus. The government may believe that if it forced HIV-positive doctors to retire, it would send the message that all HIV carriers, not just doctors, are dangerous. While the government has tried to assure the public that HIV carriers are not dangerous, the public is not convinced. But people have not made their wishes felt in Washington, because the average patient would prefer not to be worked on by an infected person. What would you do if your dentist told you he had HIV? Most people would change dentists immediately!

Chances Of Contracting HIV

The government's position is that except for the six patients in Florida, there has not been any recorded transmission of HIV from a doctor of any type to a patient; this may or may not be true. But someone or something is dangerous because the disease is spreading despite condom ads and assurances from Washington and the CDC. But we may not be as safe from exposure in other ways as we are told. The next few years will show exactly what is happening and how much at risk the majority of people in the low-risk categories are. So far, we may have simply been lucky.

The dental profession has accepted the universal precaution guidelines and individual dentists have worked to implement them into their practices. These efforts have been made at considerable cost and trouble but there has been little resistance other than complaining about heavy-handed government bureaucracies intruding into new areas. As conservative as dentists tend to be, they have accepted all the changes as necessary and perhaps long overdue.

Protecting Yourself

As a dental patient, your best way to protect yourself is to get your immune system in better condition. Ridding yourself of toxic metals is one of the best ways to achieve this protection. People who hear the truth and act on it first will be far ahead. Now is the time to get your work done by someone who knows how to do it before the big rush. Once the majority of Americans want their toxic metals removed, the demand will make it difficult to get into any dental office. Do not delay too long!

For your routine dental treatment go to a dentist who practices universal precautions. Make sure that the dentist changes gloves each time he begins to work on you. If you have any concerns about cleanliness, ask the dental assistant how equipment is sterilized. You can even ask to see the sterilization area. In one case, it was reported that a dentist who did not own a sterilizing machine admitted to lying whenever a patient asked if his instruments were sterilized. With this story in mind, as well as the fact that it is your life at stake, ask in a friendly and curious manner if you could see how the sterilization is done.

It has not been shown that going to the dentist carries a risk of contracting HIV. Other risks are real and should be addressed by each of us individually.

It is wise to cut your other risk factors by practicing "safe sex." If we faced reality and reduced the number of sex partners, we would cut the transmission rate considerably. In reality, "safe sex" is not practiced by wearing a condom but by being in a truly monogamous relationship or by being celibate.

It is easy to dismiss HIV when it happens to "them." But do not become complacent. We are all in the same boat, and there may be no way to get out. It is easy to condemn those that brought the problem on themselves, but before it is all over, compassion must overcome condemnation.

20

THE FUTURE OF DENTISTRY

If you believe the ADA press releases, you would think that Americans would soon see the end of all dental problems. For example, the ADA has released encouraging reports about a possible vaccine to prevent tooth decay every year or two. What people do not realize is that the ADA has been releasing these reports for 20 years. What the ADA does not emphasis enough is that there is something better than a vaccine available now, eating healthier and avoiding sugar!

Breakthrough Products

The advertising industry is no better than the ADA in misleading the public. Advertisers continually tell you about all the "breakthrough" dental products. For example, they now sell a toothpaste with baking soda, hydrogen peroxide, and fluoride combined. You would be better off saving your money and using inexpensive baking soda and peroxide by themselves. There are no magic products that can stop the damage we cause through our poor food choices but for some reason we still believe the advertisers' hype.

If we follow the current trend, the future of dentistry will be doing more of the same or worse. The use of tooth-damaging techniques and more toxic materials will continue unless this and other books raise enough anger among the public that the profession begins to put health above convenience. Change can only occur if helping people becomes more important to dentists than the number of crowns done each month.

Governmental Agenda

The government has its own ideas about the future of dentistry. Dentists have not yet realized what their fate will be if the government planners have their way. Fifteen years ago, a single government bureaucrat in Health and Human Services decided that if there were more dentists, the cost of dental treatment would decline. The resulting increase in the number of dentists was accomplished by offering monetary incentives to dental schools to double the size of their graduating classes. The greed motive worked fine on the dental schools because in four to five years there was a glut of dentists graduating, so many that they could not be absorbed into the dental marketplace. This glut created great hardships on the young dentists and the increase in the number of dentists did not lower the cost of dental services because fees are based on the cost of providing services, which did not drop. Instead dentists now work under more economic pressure, which means they need to do more crowns to compensate.

Eventually, the dental schools began to get pressure from alumni complaining about the problems caused by all these new dentists. The government stopped the incentives and the dental schools went back to their previous size with several schools having to close. The current number of graduating dentists is back to its 1970 level, but an excess of dentists still exists. So much for the success of bureaucratic planning. Unfortunately, the bureaucrats will always be around and will always find new ways to "improve" the future.

Managed Health Care

Traditionally, a doctor was an independent businessman who served his patients. If he did a good job, the patients would come back and if not, they would go elsewhere. He was responsive to his patients and in effect was their employee.

Under managed care the doctor is an employee of the corporately managed health care. The future of this managed care is no longer based on the doctor-patient relationship but will be controlled by insurance companies, politicians, employers, and other forces that have a financial interest. The emphasis may easily shift from healing and humanitarianism to efficiency and bottom lines. Forcing costs down to increase profits will be the reality.

While patients still have trust in doctors to act in their best interest, many signs point to more and more people becoming disenchanted with the medical care system. It will be difficult for doctors not to become representatives of their new employers, the corporate owners of the healthcare system be they hospitals, HMO's, or insurance companies. This fundamental change creates a system not unlike the government-controlled systems found in most other Western countries. Whether corporate ownership will be more successful than government control is still unknown. The loser will be the patient as pressure lowers the quality of treatment and access becomes more difficult, which will not happen right away but over the next decade or two.

As recently as June 2000, the US. Supreme Court ruled that it is acceptable for HMO doctors to withhold care even if patients are harmed. In addition, the doctors can receive bonuses for doing so. Guess whose money is used to pay those bonuses?

Managed Dental Care

The same pressures are beginning to be felt in dentistry, the major difference being that dentistry is an active profession where the dentist actually performs intricate services that are difficult to delegate. For example, when a cavity is found the dentist does not write a prescription and go on to the next patient, but actually must fix the tooth. The difficulty in performing dental procedures will slow the takeover of dentistry but it will not stop it. The pressure to join managed care dental groups will become a choice between joining or going bankrupt. Older dentists will resist and eventually, will retire. Younger dentists will have few options and accept the financial relationship offered by the corporate structure.

The new emphasis on managed dental care could result in some drastic changes in how dental services are delivered, some of which might seem like advantages to patients. For example, clinics might be open 70 hours a week, take drop-in patients and fees may be paid in part or in full by a variety of prepaid dental plans and governmental programs. Those advantages may sound good to people who think all dentists are the same and that all dental materials are safe.

The downside is that managed dental care will exert enormous economic pressure, which can lead to mediocrity. In such a setting the quality of care is not as important as quantity. The closest example of the type of care people can expect in a large clinic setting is the military dental clinics. The work done meets the standards set by the government, but it would not be the place the average person would want to go if given a choice.

Under managed dental care patients will be captives of a system designed to deliver dental services at the lowest cost. For example, a composite filling will not be approved if a mercury filling can be done at a lower cost. These changes will not happen in the future but are occurring right now.

Fundamental changes in the way dental plans are being administrated have already happened. The corporations backing managed dental care will not be willing to pay the costs involved with patients having their toxic dental materials removed. With close to half of every dollar spent on dentistry coming from some type of dental plan, the economic pressure to not change toxic dental materials already exists. If you are sick, you cannot be concerned about what the corporations want but only in what you need.

It is not to your advantage to play by their rules if it slows or stops you from getting well.

Controlling Your Dental Future

If the emphasis shifts from repair to prevention, you have an alternative. That does not mean more fluorides; it means better eating habits, particularly LESS SUGAR. This alternative emphasizes having healthy children with complete sets of whole (unfilled) teeth and a future in which the reaction would be shock if a cavity were found, followed by a complete evaluation as to why it happened. This alternative would do away with the expectation of having routine decay and a mouth full of fillings. An adult with a full set of unfilled teeth would be the rule, not a rarity.

In this scenario the costs of dentistry would be almost nothing because no treatment would be needed. That is a future worth working toward.

The best part of a future with no dental problems is that it is within your ability to have today. You control your dental future. You can accept the normal dental damage, or you can work toward a decay-free and filling-free mouth. You may already have damage, but all future damage can be stopped or minimized.

Your children and your grandchildren can benefit from your knowledge; they may be the first in your family to be free of dental damage. You need not wait until someone at the top makes the decisions for you. Any decision our leaders would make about dental health care may be driven more by money than concern about your oral health. You have the power to create your own preferred future. What will it be?

Public Awareness Is Crucial

Any person or small group that challenges the credibility of powerful organizations is usually threatened or dealt with harshly to keep them in line to maintain the status quo. Currently, the ADA threatens mercury-free dentists with loss of license, even though dental societies in other countries are abandoning mercury fillings. Therefore, before any change is possible it is critical for the general population to become involved; this is not easy to accomplish because the media are more controlled by those in power, if for no other reason than they have better access.

The Power of the Marketplace

A few years ago media attention made the general public aware of the problems with the pesticide Alar, which had been legally used on apples for years. Consumer groups had lobbied against Alar for years but were not able to stop its use until the public became involved; when they did, the results were dramatic. People immediately quit buying apples and apple products. The growers had no choice but to stop the use of Alar. People did not settle for the government's or the growers' reassurances; they just quit buying.

While Alar posed some health risks to children, it was not nearly as severe a threat as are dental materials. The same reaction from the public must happen with regard to mercury fillings and other toxic dental materials. Once enough people become concerned about dental materials as a threat to their health and the environment, there will be a flood of media attention. More and more people will learn of the problems. People will demand a call for action, refusing to allow any dentist to use these materials on them.

Once the general population becomes afraid and quits buying, the bureaucracy will act. They will not act to protect the public from mercury, but WILL ACT TO PROTECT THEMSELVES FROM THE PUBLIC. Then, the tide will quickly turn. Mercury use will stop and other problems with dental procedures and materials will be openly discussed. That day cannot come soon enough.

This book is your call to action. Tell your friends about the problems with current dental practices. Give away copies of this book. Spread the word to anyone who will listen. As soon as the critical number of concerned people is reached, the media will sense a hot story and get involved. The message will then spread to every home in a few days. Therefore, the end of the use of mercury fillings and other damaging materials and procedures depends on you, the reader. This is your opportunity to directly contribute to the health of all Americans.

APPENDIX I-Patient's Consent Form

Patient _____

I,_____(dentist),
propose to do the following treatment:
_____

I recommend this treatment because:

I will use the following materials:

The possible side effects of the treatment are:

*The possible side effects of the materials are:

The estimated cost is:

Alternative treatments are:
   1)_____
   2)_____

Signed_____(dentist)

Date_____

I have read and understood the above information and accept the above treatment as proposed.

Signed_____(patient)

Date _____

Note: This is a generic form that may or may not have any legal validity. It is offered to readers as a help in understanding their treatment options and the possible effects of those treatments. It is also to help the dentist under- stand the possible effects of their treatments on patients. By putting the information down in writing, misconceptions can be dispelled before any work is done.
   *The best way to see the negative effects of a dental material is to see the dentist's copy of the Material Safety and Data Sheet. Dentists are required by law to have a copy for every material used in their office.

APPENDIX II - DAMS

DAMS (Dental Amalgam Mercury Syndrome) is a not-for-profit group formed by people who have been damaged by mercury fillings and other dental materials. This independent group, now organized in most states and in several countries, tries to help people seeking to get rid of their mercury and works with dentists who remove mercury using the proper techniques. DAMS is concerned that people with problems from dental materials have their work done correctly to achieve the best results in reversing their health problems.

DAMS is adamant in its desire for a ban on the further use of mercury in dentistry. It is difficult to reverse problems caused by mercury fillings when they are still being placed by the millions. DAMS works through the political process that will lead to a ban because it does not believe that either the dental profession or the government agencies that should protect the public will order an end to the use of mercury unless they are forced. The group believes that change in dental practice will require political action by elected representatives under pressure from voters.

DAMS is a dedicated group whose members know from first-hand experience the damage dental materials can cause. Not only does DAMS act as a support group for people struggling to get well, but also publishes an excellent newsletter.

Information or membership can be obtained from:

DAMS
P.O. Box 7249
Minneapolis, MN 55407-0249
1-800-331-6265

APPENDIX III

Source For Compatibility Tests

Clifford Consulting and Research
PO. Box 17597
Colorado Springs, CO 80935-7597
1-719-550-0008
FAX 719-550-0009

SUGGESTED READING LIST

The Cure for All Diseases
The Cure for All Advanced
Cancers
by
Hulda R. Clark, Ph.D.
Available at:
New Century Press
1055 Bay Blvd. Suite C
Chula Vista, CA 91911
(800) 519-2465

Mercury-Free
by
Dr. James Hardy
Available at:
Access Publishers Network
1-800-507-2665

The Key to Ultimate Health
by
Ellen Brown and Richard
Hansen, D.D.S.
Available at:
Advanced Health Research
Publishing
1-888-792-1102

Root-Canal Cover-Up
"New" Nutrition
by
George Meinig, D.D.S.
Available at:
Bion Publishing
P.O. Box 10
Ojai, CA 93023-0010

It's All In Your Head
Why Raise Ugly Kids
by
Hal Huggins, D.D.S.
Available at:
M.S. Huggins Diagnostics
Center
1-800-331-2303

Whole Body
Dentistry
by
Mark Breiner,
D.D.S.
Available at:
Quantum Press
1-888-792-1102

INDEX

mercury-free..3, 4, 5, 22, 131,
157, 158, 167, 189, 235,
250, 280, 314, 428
meridian..80, 256, 257, 258,
374
metal-free..3, 270, 275, 317,
320, 321
microwaves.........136, 168
Minamata Bay..............142
molar....11, 12, 18, 19, 228,
302, 310, 311, 322, 350,
351, 372, 373
Morter, Dr. Ted..............26
multiple sclerosis..93, 101, 106,
144, 167

N

nickel..19, 131, 177, 179, 235,
254, 280, 316, 318, 328,
356, 375, 376, 383, 384,
397
NICO...........................364

O

onlay......282, 307, 310, 324
OSHA..105, 125, 126, 131,
137, 188
osteoporosis..216, 218, 222

P

partial..19, 20, 185, 294, 324,
365, 375, 376, 377, 378
periosteum........... 360, 361
pins..267, 268, 269, 270, 271
plaque.. 207, 208, 214, 215,
225, 232, 234, 243, 389,
410
post..12, 14, 15, 36, 128, 199,
265, 327, 328, 329, 338,
363
Pottenger, Dr. Francis.. 200,
201, 205
PPO.......... 84, 85, 86, 194
Price, Dr. Weston.. 43, 199,
200, 201, 202, 204, 225,
348, 371, 381
pulp chamber... 12, 14, 285,
297, 309, 312, 337, 338,
342
pulpotomy.................... 355

Q

quicksilver.................. 137

R

radioactivity............ 87, 110
recontouring.......... 285, 286
removable partial.. 294, 323,
324, 326, 375

T

U

V

W

X

Z

ORDER FORM

TOOTH TRUTH _____ copies at $21.95 each

$3.50 Shipping for one copy

_____ Additional copies @ $1.00

_____ Indiana Residents Only Total $1.15

Check____ Money Order____ MasterCard_____ Visa_____

Card#_____

Expiration Date_____

Name_____

Address_____

City_____State_____Zip_____

This book and others are available on our website:
www.dentistry-toothtruth.com

Send mail orders to: Tooth Truth
                            639 Washington Street
                            Columbus, IN 47201
Phone orders at: 1-812-376-8525

447